Basic Principles and Practice in Surgery

Edited by Miana Gabriela Pop

Published in London, United Kingdom

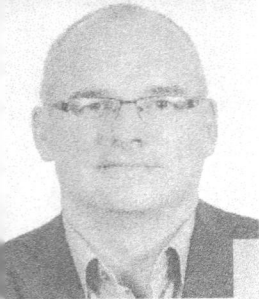
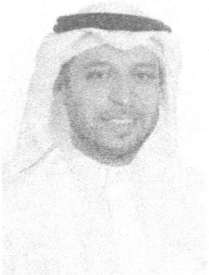
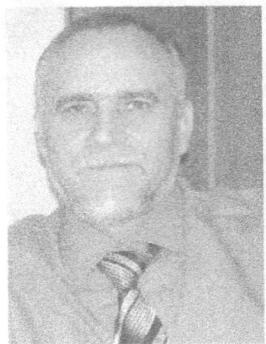
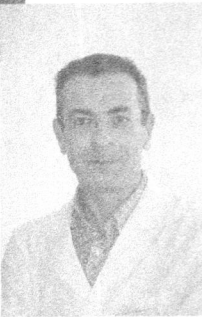
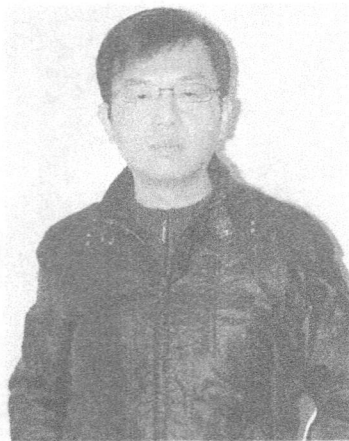
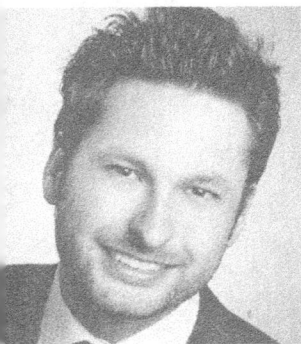
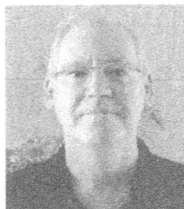

IntechOpen

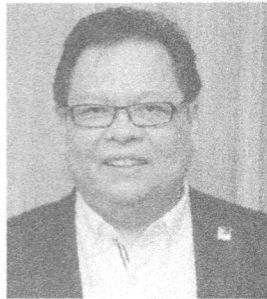
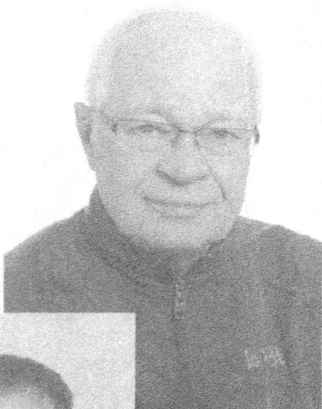
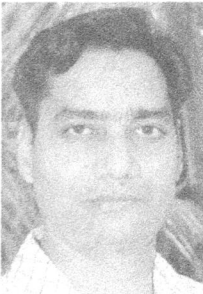
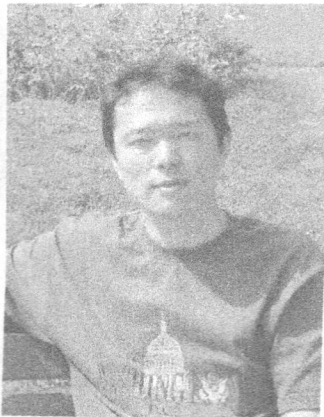
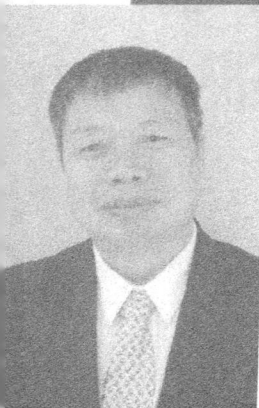
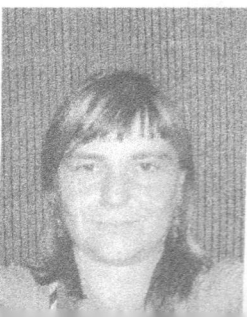

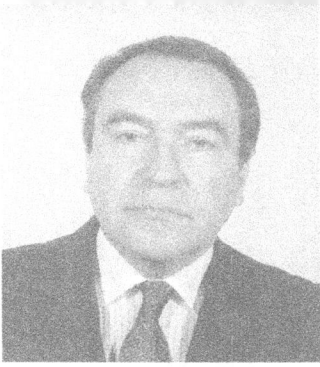

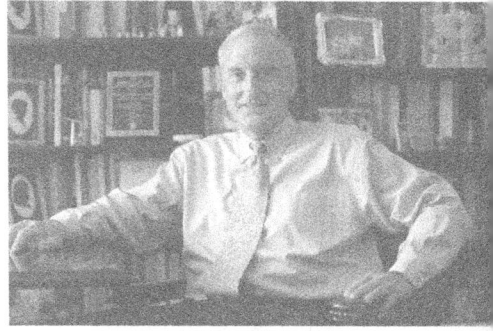

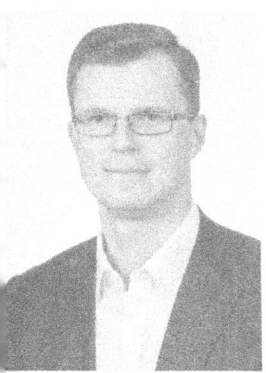

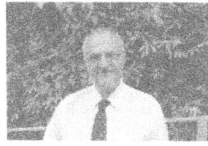

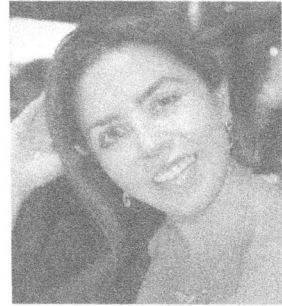

Supporting open minds since 2005

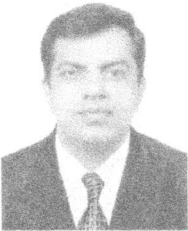

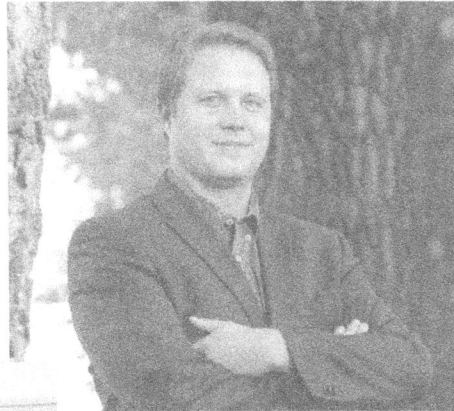

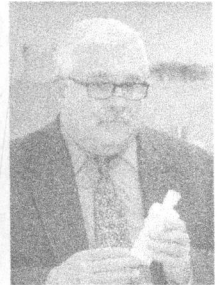

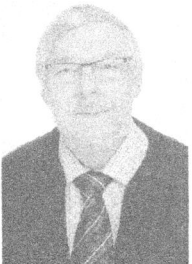

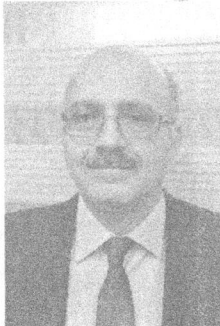

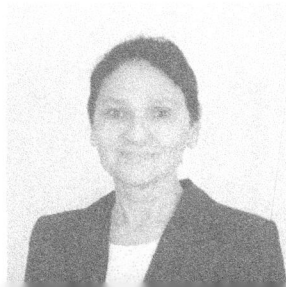

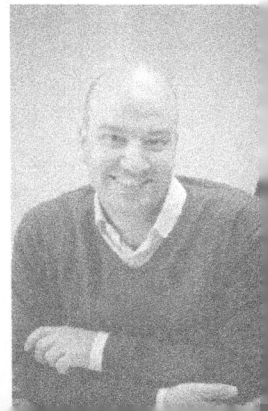

Basic Principles and Practice in Surgery
http://dx.doi.org/10.5772/intechopen.78251
Edited by Miana Gabriela Pop

Contributors
Maroun Moukarzel, Charbel Chalouhy, Bruno Costa Do Prado, Alana Puppin, Jose Tadeu Carvalho Martins, Fabiana Lima Marques, Robson Dettman Jarske, Octavio Meneghelli Galvão Gonçalves, Miana Gabriela Pop, Anca Budusan

Notice
Statements and opinions expressed in the chapters are these of the individual contributors and not necessarily those of the editors or publisher. No responsibility is accepted for the accuracy of information contained in the published chapters. The publisher assumes no responsibility for any damage or injury to persons or property arising out of the use of any materials, instructions, methods or ideas contained in the book.

First published in London, United Kingdom, 2019 by IntechOpen
IntechOpen is the global imprint of INTECHOPEN LIMITED, registered in England and Wales, registration number: 11086078, The Shard, 25th floor, 32 London Bridge Street
London, SE19SG – United Kingdom
Printed in Croatia

British Library Cataloguing-in-Publication Data
A catalogue record for this book is available from the British Library

Additional hard and PDF copies can be obtained from orders@intechopen.com

Basic Principles and Practice in Surgery
Edited by Miana Gabriela Pop
p. cm.
Print ISBN 978-1-78984-177-0
Online ISBN 978-1-78984-178-7
eBook (PDF) ISBN 978-1-83962-180-2

We are IntechOpen,
the world's leading publisher of
Open Access books
Built by scientists, for scientists

4,300+
Open access books available

116,000+
International authors and editors

130M+
Downloads

151
Countries delivered to

Our authors are among the
Top 1%
most cited scientists

12.2%
Contributors from top 500 universities

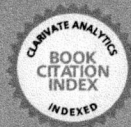

Interested in publishing with us?
Contact book.department@intechopen.com

Numbers displayed above are based on latest data collected.
For more information visit www.intechopen.com

Meet the editor

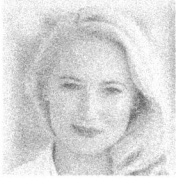

Miana Gabriela Pop was born in Cluj-Napoca, Romania, on September 3, 1988. In 2013, she graduated from the Faculty of Medicine of the „Iuliu Hatieganu" University of Medicine and Pharmacy, Cluj-Napoca, Romania. Miana-Gabriela Pop is a general surgery resident and university assistant in the Department of Anatomy and Embryology of the University of Medicine and Pharmacy „Iuliu Hatieganu," Cluj-Napoca, Romania.

Passionate about surgery, she completed her residency training through valuable professional fellowship programs in the field of hepato-bilio-pancreatic surgery and minimally invasive procedures in France (Centre Hepato-Biliare Paul Brousse, Paris, IRCAD Laparoscopic Training Center, Strasbourg) and the Netherlands (the Netherlands Cancer Institute—NKI, Amsterdam). This scientific activity has resulted in the publication of seven anatomy and surgery chapters and 11 scientific papers.

Contents

Preface

This publication aims to support young doctors and surgery residents during their training period. A surgical residency is a crucial period for a young doctor. A great volume of theoretical information along with difficult and demanding practical skills need to be acquired in a relatively short period of time. Often, we are tempted to focus on specific pathologies, complex surgical interventions, or innovative minimally invasive procedures and we skip the basic principles of a surgical act, which should be the pillar of further development. Consolidating basic notions and skills in surgery not only can help us learn and master different surgical steps and further complete interventions, but applied on time and correctly could represent a saving gesture.

In the field of surgery, significant progress has been made in the last few decades in both molecular and surgical pathology. Current research activity focuses more and more on identifying and characterizing molecules that play a role in cancer carcinogenesis, but also in finding new and effective therapeutic targets. Not least, many biomarkers have been studied in various types of cancer as predictors of advanced stages of neoplastic disease or poor overall survival, but results are not homogeneous.

This book is a tool for rapid, suitable acquisition of elementary surgical notions and techniques, which represent the basis for training today's resident to become tomorrow's surgeon.

Miana Gabriela Pop
'Iuliu Haţieganu' University of Medicine and Pharmacy,
Cluj-Napoca, Romania

Section 1

Introduction

Chapter 1

Introductory Chapter: General Surgery in the Era of Modern Molecular Biomarkers

Miana Gabriela Pop

1. Introduction

The history of surgery begins in antiquity, when various maneuvers were performed in order to treat injury and wounds. The results of these procedures were mostly characterized by increased rates of massive bleeding and severe infectious complications. An important role in surgery progress at that time has been the development of varied instruments which have begun to be used more and more in surgical practice. Initially characterized by elevated rates of postoperative mortality, surgery developed furthermore after the introduction, at the end of the nineteenth century, of aseptic and antiseptic methods.

Claudius Galen (129–200 AD) introduces for the first time the use of catgut for surgical sutures. Galen also made important contributions in the field of anatomy; he was the first to describe the anatomy of the recurrent laryngeal nerve [1]. Moreover, he demonstrated their importance in phonetics by cutting, in front of an auditory in Rome, the recurrent laryngeal nerves of a pig that remained afterward mute [1].

The first successful open appendectomy of an 11-year-old boy was reported, back in 1735, by Claudius Aymand (1681–1740), while the first laparoscopic removal of the appendix was realized in 1981 by Kurt Semm [2]. For years after, the gallbladder was removed for the first time through laparoscopy [3]. Before the introduction of laparoscopic techniques as a treatment option in various human pathologies, a large number of experimental interventions were performed on animals. Georg Kelling was the promoter of this learning technique, most of his experimental studies being performed on dogs [4]. The first laparoscopic intervention was performed on a human in 1910 by Hans Christian Jacobaeus and consisted of a "laparothoracoscopy" [5].

Due to the enthusiasm in terms of implementation of minimally invasive surgical techniques, natural orifice transluminal endoscopic surgery (NOTES) has been further developed. In 2004, the team lead by Dr. Kallo at the Johns Hopkins University reported the first NOTES procedure and demonstrated the feasibility of intra-abdominal exploration through the use of an endoscope [6]. Since then, the hybrid techniques have been developed as a combined endoscopic and laparoscopic approach [7].

After the revolution of laparoscopic procedures, robotic-assisted surgery was introduced in 1983, along with increasing interest in virtual reality [8]. Currently, there are several types of robotic systems (AESOP, EndoAssist, Neuromate, da Vinci, PROBOT (surgeon robot for prostatectomies), PAKY (robotic system for percutaneous access)), each with its advantages and disadvantages [8]. Some of the main advantages of robotic surgery are better three-dimensional (3D) vision and better ergonomics; the removal of psychological tremor while increase costs would represent the main disadvantage [9].

The use of ultrasound in surgery or so-called interventional ultrasound has started in the 1960s and has been of great interest since then, developed in various directions such as liver and pancreatic surgery and surgery of the biliary tract but also in cardiovascular surgery and neurosurgery [10]. Even if its importance in intraoperative guidance, accurate diagnosis, and decision-making has been demonstrated, no specific training programs in residency curriculum have been established so far [11].

Indocyanine green (ICG) absorbs near-infrared light and through this mechanism allows for an accurate identification of the vascularization of different organs and tissues [12]. First used in cardiology to measure cardiac output and in ophthalmology to study in detail retinal vessels, in laparoscopic surgery ICG was used as a mean to improve vision [13]. Fluorescence-image-guided surgery (FISG) has been used in sentinel lymph node identification, in neurosurgery, or for neuroendocrine tumor detection. Moreover, the use of ICG in surgery has been shown to intervene in establishing the demarcation limit for surgical resection [12].

Development of mentoring programs through the use of telemedicine could be of great interest in the future from several points of view. First, by addressing this method, the difficulty in providing health care to people from disadvantage areas that do not have access to specialized, healthcare institutions could be overcome [14]. Moreover, a highly specialized level of surgical act could be offered by surgeons with less experience in a particular field. Not least, telementoring could represent an important pylon of surgical training programs and development of surgical techniques.

Through the identification of various biomarkers in cancer pathology, the concept of personalized medical and surgical treatment will be applied more and more in the future. Starting from this concept, patient treatment will need to be applied individually, depending on the molecular characteristics of the tumors. Surgical treatment will not represent a standardized procedure but one centered on patient needs and on its peculiarities.

For personalized surgery, 3D systems and the virtual surgical planning are important tools whose applicability are to be tested in the future more and more. The main advantage of these procedures consists in their ability to reproduce, with high accuracy, and patient's anatomic characteristics and possible variants of a specific organ vasculature; this aspect allows improvement of the surgical procedure due to preoperative assessment of the surgical and technical plan to be applied [15]. So far, 3D systems and virtual surgical planning were mostly used in craniofacial surgery [15, 16].

All in all, there is a tremendous progress in the field of general surgery from its beginnings to the present. Efforts should be made to apply and develop modern available techniques in order to constantly improve surgical outcome and patient benefits.

Conflict of interest

No conflict of interest to declare.

Author details

Miana Gabriela Pop
Iuliu Hațieganu University of Medicine and Pharmacy, Cluj-Napoca, Romania

*Address all correspondence to: miana_my@yahoo.com

IntechOpen

References

[1] Stathopoulos P. Galen s contribution to head and neck surgery. Journal of Oral and Maxillofacial Surgery. 2017;**75**(6):1095-1096

[2] Meljnikov I, Radojcic B, Grebeldinger S, Radojcic N. History of surgical treatment of appendicitis. Medicinski Pregled. 2009;**62**(9-10):489-492

[3] Blum CA, Adams DB. Who did the first laparoscopic cholecystectomy? Journal of Minimal Access Surgery. 2011;7(3):165-168

[4] Hatzinger M, Fesenko A, Sohn M. The first human laparoscopy and NOTES operation: Dimitrij oscarovic ott (1855-1929). Urologia Internationalis. 2014;**92**(4):387-391

[5] Kelley WE. The Evolution of laparoscopy and the revolution in surgery in the decade of the 1990s. Journal of the Society of Laparoendoscopic Surgeons. 2008;**12**(4):351-357

[6] Kallo AN, Singh VK, Jagannath SB, Niiyama H, et al. Flexible transgastric peritoneoscopy: A novel approach to diagnosis and therapeutic interventions in the peritoneal cavity. Gastrointestinal Endoscopy. 2004;**60**:114-117

[7] Bernhardt J, Sasse S, Ludwig K, Meier PN. Update in natural orifice transluminal endoscopic surgery (NOTES). Current Opinion in Gastroenterology. 2017;**33**(5):346-351

[8] Otero JR, Paparel P, Atreya D, Touijer K, Guilonneau B. History, evolution and application of robotic surgery in urology. Urology Robotic Surgery. 2007;**60**(4):335-341

[9] Schreuder HWR, Verheijen RHM. Robotic surgery. BJOG: An International Journal of Obstetrics & Gynaecology. 2009;**116**(2):198-213

[10] Makuuchi M, Torzili G, Machi J. History of intraoperative ultrasound. Ultrasound in Medicine & Biology. 1998;**24**(9):1229-1242

[11] Beal EW, Sigmond BR, Sage-Silski L, Lahey S, Nguyen V, Bahmer DP. Point-of-care ultrasound in general surgery residency training. Journal of Ultrasound in Medicine. 2017;**36**(12):2577-2584. DOI: 10.1002/jum/14298

[12] Ferroni MC, Sentell K, Abaza R. Current role and indications for the use of indocyanine green in robot-assisted urologic surgery. European Urology Focus. 2018;**4**:648-651. DOI: 10.1016/j.euf.2018.07009

[13] Boni L, David G, Mangano A, Dionigi G, Rausei S, Spampatti S, et al. Clinical applications of indocyanine green (ICG) enhanced fluorescence in laparoscopic surgery. Surgical Endoscopy. 2014;**29**(7):2046-2055

[14] El-Sabawi B, Magee W. The evolution of surgical telementoring: Current applications and future directions. Annals of Translational Medicine. 2016;**4**(20):391. DOI: 10.21037/atm.2016.10.04

[15] Efanov JI, Roy AA, Huang KN, Borsuk DE. Virtual surgical planning: The pearls and pitfalls. Plastic and Reconstructive Surgery. Global Open. 2018;**6**(1):e1443

[16] Yu H, Shen SG. Virtual surgical planning in the treatment of facial asymmetry. Oral and Maxillofacial Surgery. 2017;**46**(1):172

Section 2

Molecular Surgical Pathology

Chapter 2

Stem Cell Markers in Colon Cancer

Miana Gabriela Pop

Abstract

Colon cancer incidence is increasing in young people. Even if, so far, colon cancer had a maximum incidence in the sixth and seventh decades of life, lately its incidence in people age 50 and younger is increasing. Thus, colon cancer still represents a major health problem despite constant research made in the field. Early detection of colon cancer is mandatory for an appropriate treatment of the disease and to attain increased overall survival. Even if various stem cell markers have been studied in order to evaluate their prognostic value in colon cancer cases, results in literature are heterogeneous, and no clear consensus has been drafted so far. This paper aims to review the most important stem cell markers identified in colon cancer and to establish their role in both cancer diagnosis and progression.

Keywords: colon, cancer, stem cell markers, CD133, CD44, CD166, EpCAM

1. Introduction

Colon cancer is a frequent neoplastic disease which is ranked second in female after breast cancer and third in men after prostate and lung and cancer [1]. Despite constant research in the field of colon cancer, its incidence continues to be high worldwide. Moreover, the number of people age 50 or younger diagnosed with colon cancer is dramatically increasing in last years. This finding upholds the idea that colon cancer is not a disease considered to be under control at this time, and efforts should be made in order to better understand its pathogenic mechanism.

Five-year overall survival in colon cancer ranges from 90% in early stages to less than 10% in advanced, metastatic cases [2]. It is thus important to try to diagnose the disease in early stage, so an appropriate treatment can be applied. Achieving this condition can be difficult, considering the fact that a large number of colon cancer patients present with late stage, often inoperable tumors.

Even if important progress has been made in terms of imaging diagnosis of colon cancer, early detection is still difficult to achieve. An important role in detecting early colon cancer cases is assigned to screening programs that have to be applied nationally, and population should be well informed of their importance. More than detecting incipient cases, early detection of advanced cases is also of crucial importance, and efforts should continue in this direction by further research groups.

Colon cancer stem cells (CCSCs) are multipotent neoplastic cells that have the ability to differentiate and initiate the carcinogenesis process [3]. Due to their increased viability, CCSCs are responsible for both tumor growth and tumor recurrence [4, 5]. According to a recent study, the presence of CCSCs is also responsible for resistance to chemotherapeutic treatments, which is observed in some cases [5]. A new treatment concept linked to CCSCs is based on their early detection, before the onset of the tumor, which would allow them to target with apoptotic substances.

Detection of cancer stem cells (CSCs) in various digestive and extra-digestive cancers has been a topic of great interest in the literature of recent years and was frequently done using cluster of differentiation (CD) markers. In colon cancer, various biomarkers have been identified at the surface of CSCs, and their role in colon cancer is currently being tested: EpCAM, CD133, CD29, CD24, CD44, CD166, ALDH1A1, and ALDH1B1 [3, 4].

The aim of this paper is to review the most important biomarkers which have been identified in colon cancer, to expose current information regarding their role in colon cancer development and progression and to identify possible predictive biomarkers for advanced stages of the disease.

2. CD133/prominin-1

CD133 was first described in 1997 by Yin et al. on the cellular surface of hematopoietic cells [6]. Also called prominin-1, CD133 is a 5-transmembranaire glycoprotein of 120 kDa which can be found in two isoforms: CD133-1 and CD133-2 [5–7]. CD133 is found on the short arm of chromosome 4 [5]. Its cellular function is unclear [5–7], but its involvement in cell-cell and cell-matrix interactions was described [5]. According to some recent studies, CD133 expression is an important tool in cancer stem cells (CSCs) identification and characterization [7]. CD133 was found to be expressed in various digestive (pancreatic, liver, colorectal) and non-digestive tumors (brain, kidney, prostate, ovary cancer) [7–9]. CD133 expression promotes cancer cell proliferation through activation of Wnt/beta-catenin pathway [10, 11]. Moreover, in highly expression CD133 cancer stem cells, the development of solid tumor mass is assured by the anti-apoptotic factors BCL-2, BCL-XL, and MCL-1 that are stimulated through PI3K pathway, with subsequent activation of Akt [11]. Even if various studies focused on targeting CSCs and especially CD133 due to its overexpression, most of the results arise from in vitro research and not from clinical experience. Targeted therapy was tested using Anti-CD133 scFv immunotoxins by Waldron et al. that found an interruption of the protein synthesis secondary to this process [12].

CD133 expression in colon cancer was confirmed 10 years after its initial description in 2007 [13, 14], when Obrien et al. proved that neoplastic cells expressing CD133 have the ability to form solid colon cancer masses in immunodeficient mice. From that point, many studies focused on CD133 expression in colon cancer carcinogenesis. Various studies analyzed CD133 expression in relation to clinical and pathological characteristics of the neoplastic patients, but result were inconsistent. CD133 expression correlates with the degree of tumor wall involvement (T) [15], with distant metastasis formation (M) [5, 16], with venous (V) and lymphatic (L) invasion [15]. A relation between CD133 expression and tumor recurrence was also noticed in one study [5], while other research groups found a significant association between CD133 expression and tumor size [7]. CD133 expression was correlated in some studies with a poor degree of tumor differentiation (G) [7], but the result was not confirmed by other studies where CD133 expression was found more frequent in moderate (G2) and well differentiated (G1) colon tumor tissues [17].

Chemoresistance was also found to be influenced by CD133 expression in colon cancer especially due to upregulation of FLICE-like inhibitory protein (FLIP), a ligand that inhibits tumor necrosis factors (TNF)-mediated apoptosis [11]. According to some studies, tumors expressing CD133 are more likely to be resistant to chemotherapy [5, 7, 18]. Moreover, tumors expressing high CD133 and CD44 biomarkers on the cellular surface are expected to be unresponsive to chemotherapy when compared to tumors where the expression of the two molecules is low or absent [16].

Results are contradictory in terms of CD133 expression in liver metastases secondary to colon cancer. While CD133 expression in liver metastases was thought to predict a better overall survival (OS) in colon cancer patients [19], Spelt et al. found, in a recent study, different results [4]. According to them, CD133 expression in liver metastases is associated with worse overall survival (OS). Results in favor of a worse prognostic impact of CD133 expression in liver metastases are suggested also by Narita et al. which demonstrated an increased CD133 expression in cases of early recurrence of liver metastases compared with a low CD133 expression in late recurrent liver metastases [20].

In terms of survival, overexpression of CD133 was associated with worse overall survival in some studies [16, 21–23] and also with low disease-free survival interval [23], but the relation was not found by others [4, 5, 17, 24, 25]. According to two recent meta-analyses, CD133 expression represents a negative prognostic factor in colon cancer patients [23, 26].

Heterogeneous results exist in literature considering CD133 role in colon cancer. Its involvement in tumor progression and metastasis formation is suggested, but its precise role remains unclear. CD133 represents a useful tool for CSCs identification and characterization in colon cancer samples. Various studies analyzed the correlation between CD133 expression and clinical and pathological characteristic of the patient, but a direct association between its degree of expression and advanced tumor stages was not confirmed. Moreover, its prognostic role regarding overall survival in colon cancer is still debated, and further studies are needed for a better characterization of the molecule in relation to colon cancer patients.

3. CD44 in colon cancer

CD44 is a type 1, 85–200 kDa transmembrane glycoprotein expressed in both normal and tumor tissues [16, 27, 28]. Discovered initially as a receptor for hyaluronic acid, the molecule has retained its affinity for it and for other components like collagens, osteopontin, or type I metalloproteinase [3, 27]. Supplementary, an adhesion function was highlighted for CD44 that was found to intervene in both cell-cell and cell-matrix interactions [4, 16]. From a structural point of view, CD44 has three main domains: an extracellular one, a transmembrane and, respectively, an intracellular domain [27]. CD44 has the capacity to present in various isoform, depending on the exons that attach to the extracellular part (CD44v) [27]. Its encoded gene is located on the short arm of chromosome 13 [29].

CD44 is expressed ubiquitary in normal tissue and participates, through lymphocytes activation, in various inflammatory processes [3, 27]; its involvement in wound healing processes was also described by some authors [3]. In neoplastic lesions, CD44 is expressed, in different isoforms, in pancreatic (CD44v8–10) and colon cancer (CD44v6) [27], in prostatic tumors (CD44s—standard isoform), in breast cancer [27], and also in epithelial ovarian cancers [30]. Through its adhesiveness properties, CD44 was found to intervene in tumor growth [16, 17]. Additionally, tumor cells expressing CD44 present with invasiveness properties and are also characterized by the capacity to initiate the metastatic process [28, 31] intervening thus in cell differentiation, proliferation, and migration [32]. The mechanisms by which the molecule intervenes in these processes remain, however, unknown, and further studies have to be performed.

Assessment of the prognostic value of CD44 was analyzed in recent papers that highlighted an association between CD44 expression and both advanced tumor stages and liver metastasis formation [27, 31]. Overexpression of CD44 in colon cancer samples was found to negatively influence overall survival of colon cancer patients [33, 34]; one study group found a negative association between CD44 expression and poor overall survival only for a specific variant of CD44 and, respectively, Cd44v2 [35]. The association between upregulation of CD44 in colon cancer and worse overall survival was not confirmed by other study groups [24, 36], but the analysis was completed based on standard isoform of CD44 (CD44s). CD44 usage as an independent prognostic factor in colon cancer patients is not currently recommended [17], but further studies need to concentrate on specific isoforms, like the one abovementioned, in order to correctly identify its value as a prognostic marker.

CD44 targeting is currently being tested in various digestive (stomach, colon cancer) [31, 37] and non-digestive cancer (lung, breast cancer) [38]. The results in terms of cancer stem cell apoptosis for in vitro and preclinical animal models are promising. In pancreatic cancer the anti-CD44 antibody tested against CD44v6 isoforms with promising antitumor results was bivatuzumab [37], while the first humanized antibody directed toward solid tumors expressing CD44 approved for clinical research is RO5429083 (NCT01358903), and the publication of results is in progress.

4. CD24 in colon cancer

CD24 is a glycoprotein located on the external surface of the cellular membrane [16]. It is formed of 27 amino acids, and it has a molecular weight of 24–70 kDa [5, 26]. Its expression was confirmed in normal nervous tissue [16] and in cancers of the colon [5], pancreas [24], breast, and prostate [26]. CD24 is involved in cellular signaling processes, in cellular differentiation, and in proliferation and is being considered a significant marker of cancer stem cells (CSCs) [4, 16, 39]. The mechanism by which CD24 participates in signaling processes seems to be related to mitogen-activated protein kinase (MAPK) and serine/threonine pathway [26].

In colon cancer, CD24 was found to be expressed in a percentage of 50–68% [24, 40]. CD44 is involved in first steps of carcinogenesis and plays an important role in liver metastasis formation [4, 9, 41–43]. Yeo et al. found CD24 a useful diagnostic marker of early colon cancer [39], whereas its expression was higher in malignant polyps than CD24 expression in colon adenomatous lesions.

No correlation was found between CD24 expression in colon cancer and tumor type or degree of differentiation (G) [5, 44]; other authors have highlighted, however, an inverse relation between CD24 expression and tumor size, poor differentiated cancers, and advanced TNM stages [39]. Regarding lymph node involvement and CD24 expression, as association between high CD24 expression and a larger number of lymph nodes involved was reported in some research papers [45] but not in others [5, 24]. In terms of overall survival, CD24 expression was in general associated with worse survival rates [16, 26]; results were not confirmed by other recent research papers [5, 24, 44]. Resistance to chemotherapeutic treatment was also objective by Nosrati et al. [5] probably due to their capacity to induce the epithelial-mesenchymal transition (EMT) mechanism [46]. Moreover, colon cancer stem cells expressing both CD133 and CD24 markers were found to be resistant to chemotherapeutic regiments based on 5-FU [47].

CD24 was highly studied in colon cancer samples, but consistent results have failed to establish its precise role in colon cancer, considering the heterogeneous results observed.

5. Epithelial cell adhesion molecule (EpCAM)

Epithelial cell adhesion molecule (EpCAM) is a Ca^{2+} independent, type I transmembrane glycoprotein with a molecular weight of 40 kDa [48] located on the basolateral surface of epithelial tissues [49]. EpCAM expression was not seen in mesenchymal or lymphoid tissues [50]. EpCAM presents with two main domains: EpICD, an intracellular domain, and EpEx, an extracellular domain of 26, respectively, and 242 amino acids [48, 51].

EpCAM was found to be overexpressed in various digestive (stomach, colon, pancreas, and esophagus) and non-digestive (prostate, ovary, breast) cancers [49]. EpCAM is principally involved in adhesion processes, but its role in cellular differentiation and progression was also confirmed [50].

A high percentage of colon cancer cases (79–99.7%) is characterized by overexpression of EpCAM molecule at tumor level [52, 53]. Moreover, EpCAM was found to be expressed also in liver metastases secondary to colon cancer, a situation that confirmed its involvement in cancer progression as well [50, 52]. Normal liver parenchyma does not express EpCAM [54].

Overexpression of EpCAM in colon cancer correlates in some studies with advanced stages of the disease [50, 55, 56], with a higher risk of metastases [55, 56], with poor differentiated (G3) patterns [54–57], with the number of lymph nodes involved (N) [48, 54], and with perilymphatic (L) and perivenous (V) invasion [54, 57] but also with worse overall survival [55, 56]. The results were not, however, confirmed by other study groups, so the predictive value of EpCAM in colon cancer patients was difficult to establish [58].

EpCAM is also involved in epithelial-mesenchymal transition (EMT) process [56]. During EMT, neoplastic cell detaches from the primary tumor (due to loss of EpCAM expression and less intercellular adhesions) to enter the lymphatic and vascular system and initiate the carcinogenesis process [56]. Detached cells, also called circulating tumor cells (CTCs), can be identified from blood samples through "liquid biopsy" technique that is based also on EpCAM detection using specific anti-EpCAM antibodies [59, 60].

In order to achieve distant metastasis formation, circulating tumor cells have to undergo a second, reversed process called mesenchymal-epithelial transition (MET) during which an upregulation of EpCAM expression at the cellular surface has been observed [59]. Secondary to it, cells acquire adhesion properties that allow them to form a solid metastatic mass [59].

Despite constant research in the field of cancer stem cell biomarkers in colon cancer, specific factors or local conditions that initiate and promote EMT or MET are insufficiently known, and further research have to be performed.

6. CD166 or ALCAM

CD166, also called activated leukocyte cell adhesion molecule (ALCAM), is a 110 kDa, transmembrane type-1 glycoprotein used for colon cancer stem cell (CCSC) identification [3, 61, 62]. Providing the leukocyte receptor function, CD166 expression was identified in both normal and colonic tissue, in the latter cases the expression being superior [3, 63]. CD166 expression in colon cancer varies between 58.6 and 76% [64, 65] and is higher in colonic adenomas [66], suggesting its involvement in colon carcinogenesis. Due to its adhesive properties, CD166 is considered to be involved in colon cancer tumor growth [62]. CD166 expression was also confirmed in pancreatic, esophageal and gastric, prostate, melanoma, and breast cancers [63].

Expression of CD166 in colon cancer was studied in relation to tumor stage [61, 64, 65], lymph node involvement [61, 64], or degree of cellular differentiation (G) [61], but even if overexpression was confirmed, no statistic significant correlation was found. Regarding overall survival of colon cancer patients, overexpression of CD166 failed to predict its outcome. Some literature studies found a worse overall survival in colon cancer cases characterized by high CD166 expression [64]. Levin et al. found that even the survival was reduced by 15 months for patients who presented colon tumors characterized by high CD166 expression compared with tumors with low or absent CD166 expression [67]. Other studies could not establish the prognostic relation of CD166 in colon cancer patients [65].

Limited number of studies analyzed CD166 expression in colon cancer patients, and existing results are inconclusive. Therefore, the role of CD166 in colon cancer remains unclear.

7. CD29

Through CD29 molecule, also known as integrin β1, cells adhere to extracellular compartment proteins and facilitate intracellular transmission of the cellular signal [68]. CD29 presents with 3 structural domains, the extracellular one being best represented [69].

Expression of CD29 was observed in normal and tumor colonic tissues, and a presumptive role in cellular differentiation was attributed to it, due to the activation of Erk signaling pathway [68, 69]. In normal colonic mucosa, CD29 is expressed in the lower part of the intestinal crypt [69] and is considered to be involved in intestinal proliferation [68]. However, its precise role in colon cancer is unknown [68].

At present, CD29 expression in colon cancer is only used as diagnostic marker for CSCs. Further studies are needed to evaluate its involvement in cancer progression and metastasis.

8. Lgr5

Leucine-rich repeat-containing G-protein coupled receptor 5 or Gpr49 is a receptor formed by eight main domains [69]. Lgr5 was identified on the cellular surface of intestinal and colonic stem cells and is being considered thus a biomarker of them [70]. Lgr5 overexpression was also confirmed in esophageal and colon cancer, in hepatocellular carcinoma, and in ovarian cancer [70].

Lgr5 is expressed in both normal and tumor colonic tissues [69]. In normal colon tissue, Lgr5 is expressed in a small area of the intestinal crypts. Its expression area increases with cell transformation in adenoma and is most elevated in colon adenocarcinoma [69]. The percentage of colon cancer patients expressing Lgr5 is, according to literature studies, around 80% [70, 71].

Overexpression of Lgr5 in colon cancer correlates with advanced stages of the disease [70, 71], with lymph node involvement (L) [70, 71] and perineural invasion [71] and distant metastases (M) [70]. Lgr5 involvement in cellular proliferation is also suggested due to the correlation found between Lgr5 expression and Ki-67 expression [70].

Lgr5 is thus considered to have a role in colon cancer development and progression and possibly in liver metastases formation as well [69]. Moreover, Lgr5 is considered to have a clinical role in predicting advanced pathological stages of colon cancer tumors [72].

9. ALDH1

Aldehyde dehydrogenase 1 is a detoxifying enzyme involved in colon cancer proliferation [73]. Expressed in low percentage in normal colonic mucosa, ALDH1 was found to be overexpressed in colon adenocarcinoma [73, 74]. A number of 75.5–76.5% of colon cancer cases express ALDH1 at tumoral level [73, 74].

ALDH1 expression is associated with colon cancer location [73], with advanced stages of the disease [75], with number of lymph nodes involved (N) [73, 75, 76], and with perivenous invasion (V) [73] but also with local tumor recurrence [75]. The association between ALDH1 expression and lymph node involvement was not seen by Zhou et al. [74].

Recently, ALDH1 expression was found to be involved in epithelial-mesenchymal transition (EMT) and could play, thus, a role in cancer progression and distant metastases formation [75–77].

Moreover, ALDH1 associates with resistance to chemotherapy [75] and poor overall survival [75, 76, 78].

In conclusion, ALDH1 could represent a promising prognostic marker in colon cancer patients that associate with advanced colon cancer stages and worse overall prognosis.

10. Conclusions

Colon cancer stem cells (CCSCs) could be responsible for tumor metastases, resistance to chemotherapy, and recurrence, and their identification is thus of major importance. However, the amount of biomarkers identified at the cellular surface of CCSC failed to become valuable prognostic markers, and further studies are necessary to evaluate their role in cancer progression and distant metastases formation.

Conflict of interest

The author declares that she has no conflict of interest.

Author details

Miana Gabriela Pop
Iuliu Hațieganu University of Medicine and Pharmacy, Cluj-Napoca, Romania

*Address all correspondence to: miana_my@yahoo.com

IntechOpen

References

[1] Ferlay J, Soerjomataram I, Dikshit R, et al. Cancer incidence and mortality worldwide: Sources, methods and major patterns in Globocan. International Journal of Cancer. 2012;**136**(5):E359-E386

[2] Coopede F, Lopomo A, Spisni R, Migliore L. Genetic and epigenetic biomarkers for diagnosis, prognosis and treatment of colorectal cancer. World Journal of Gastroenterology. 2014;**20**:943-956

[3] Ribeiro KB, da Silva ZJ, Ribeiro-Silva A, Rapatoni L, de Oliveira HF, da Cunha Tirapelli DP, et al. KRAS mutation associated with CD44/CD166 immunoexpression as predictors of worse outcome in metastatic colon cancer. Cancer Biomarkers. 2016;**16**(4):513-521

[4] Spelt L, Sasor A, Ansari D, Hilmersson KS, Andersson R. The prognostic role of cancer stem cell markers for long-term outcome after resection of colonic liver metastases. Anticancer Research. 2018;**38**(1):313-320

[5] Nosrati A, Naghshvar F, Maleki I, Salehi F. Cancer stem cells CD133 and CD24 in colorectal cancers in Northern Iran. Gastroenterology and Hepatology from Bed to Bench. 2016;**9**(2):132-139

[6] Yin AH, Miraglia S, Zanjani ED, Almeida-Porada G, Ogawa M, Leary AG, et al. AC133, a novel marker for human hematopoietic stem and progenitor cells. Blood. 1997;**90**:5002-5012

[7] Kazama S, Kishikawa J, Kiyomatsu T, Kawai K, Nozawa H, Ishihara S, et al. Expression of the stem cell marker CD133 is related to tumor development in colorectal carcinogenesis. Asian Journal of Surgery. 2018;**41**(3):274-278

[8] Pop MG, Fit AM, Bartos D, Vesa SC, Puia IC, Al-Hajjar N, et al. CD133 expression in colon cancer. An immunohistochemical analysis of 72 cases. Medicine and Pharmacy Reports. 2019;**92**(supplement 1):S60

[9] Ren F, Sheng WQ, Du X. CD133: A cancer stem cell marker, is used in colorectal cancers. World Journal of Gastroenterology. 2013;**19**:2603-2611

[10] Schmohl JU, Vallera DA. CD133, selectively targeting the root of Cancer. Toxins (Basel). 2016;**8**(6):165

[11] Barzegar Behrooz A, Syahir A, Ahmad S. CD133: Beyond a cancer stem cell biomarker. Journal of Drug Targeting. 2018;**17**:1-13

[12] Waldron NN. Development and characterization of CD133 positive cancer stem cell targeted toxins for use in carcinoma therapy [thesis]. Daniel A Vallera, University of Minnesota; 2013

[13] Obrien CA, Pollett A, Gallinger S, Dick JE. A human colon cancer cell capable of initiating tumour growth in immunodeficient mice. Nature. 2007;**445**:106-110

[14] Ricci-Vitiani L, Lombardi DG, Pilozzi E, et al. Identification and expansion of human colon-cancer-initiating cells. Nature. 2007;**445**:111-115

[15] Huang R, Mo D, Wu J, Ai H, Lu Y. CD133 expression correlates with clinicopathologic features and poor prognosis of colorectal cancer patients: An updated meta-analysis of 37 studies. Medicine. 2018;**97**(23):e10446

[16] Sahlberg SH, Spielberg D, Glimelius B, Stenerlow B, Nestor M. Evaluation of cancer stem cell markers CD133, CD44, CD24: Association with AKT isoforms and radiation resistance in colon cancer cells. PLoS One. 2014;**23**(9):e94621

[17] Pitule P, Miroslava C, Daum O, Vojtisek J, Vycital O, Hosek P, et al.

Immunohistochemical detection of cancer stem cell related markers CD44 and CD 133 in metastatic colorectal cancer patients. BioMed Research International. 2014;**2014**:7. Article ID: 432139. https://doi.org/10.1155/2014/432139

[18] Ong CW, Kim LG, Kong HH, Low LY, Iacopetta B, Soong R, et al. CD133 expression predicts for non-response to chemotherapy in colorectal cancer. Modern Pathology. 2010;**23**:450-457

[19] Yamamoto S, Tanaka K, Takeda K, Akiyama H, Ichikawa Y, Nagashima Y, et al. Patients with CD133-negative colorectal liver metastsis have a poor prognosis after hepatectomy. Annals of Surgical Oncology. 2014;**21**:1853-1861

[20] Narita M, Oussoultzoglu E, Chenard MP, Fuchshuber P, Yammamoto T, Addeo P, et al. Predicting early intrahepatic recurrence after curative resection of colorectal liver metastases with molecular markers. World Journal of Surgery. 2015;**39**:1167-1176

[21] Kemper K, Versloot M, Cameron K, Colak S, de Sousa e Melo F, de Jong JH, et al. Mutations in the Ras-Raf axis underline the prognostic value of CD133 in colorectal cancer. Clinical Cancer Research. 2012;**18**:3132-3141

[22] Saigusa S, Tanaka K, Toiyama Y, Yokoe T, Okugawa Y, Koike Y, et al. Clinical significance of CD133 and hypoxia inducible factor-1 alpha gene expression in rectal cancer after preoperative chemoradiotherapy. Clinical Oncology. 2011;**23**:323-332

[23] Chen S, Song X, Chen Z. CD133 expression and the prognosis of colorectal cancer: A systematic review and meta-analysis. PLoS One. 2013;**8**:e56380

[24] Choi D, Lee HW, Hur KY, Kim JJ, Park GS, Jang SH, et al. Cancer stem cell markers CD133 and CD24 correlate with invasiveness and differentiation in colorectal adenocarcinoma. World Journal of Gastroenterology. 2009;**15**:2258-2264

[25] Gazzaniga P, Gardilone A, Petracca A, Nicolazzo C, Raimondi C, Iacovelli R, et al. Molecular markers in circulating tumour cells from metastatic colorectal cancer patients. Journal of Cellular and Molecular Medicine. 2010;**14**:2073-2077

[26] Wang K, Xu J, Zhang J, Huang J. Prognostic role of CD133 expression in colorectal cancer: A meta-analysis. BMC Cancer. 2012;**12**:53

[27] Senbanjo LT, Chellaiah MA. CD44: A multifunctional cell surface adhesion receptor is a regulator of progression and metastasis of cancer cells. Frontiers in Cell and Development Biology. 2017;**5**:18. DOI: 10.3389/fcell.2017.00018

[28] Basakran NS. CD44 as a potential diagnostic tumor marker. Saudi Medical Journal. 2015;**36**:273-279

[29] Underhill C. CD44: The hyaluronan receptor. Journal of Cell Science. 1992;**103**(2):293-298

[30] Sillanpaa S, Anttila MA, Voutilainen K, Tammi RH, Tammi MI, Saarikoski SV, et al. CD44 expression indicated favorable prognosis in epithelial ovarian cancer. Clinical Cancer Research. 2003;**9**(14):5318-5324

[31] Todaro M, Gaggianesi M, Catalano V, Benfante A, Iovino F, Biffoni M, et al. Cd44v6 is a marker of constitutive and reprogrammed cancer stem cell driving colon cancer metastasis. Cell Stem Cell. 2014;**14**(3):342-356

[32] Yan Y, Zuo X, Wei D. Concise review: Emerging role of CD44 in cancer stem cells: A promising biomarker and therapeutic target. Stem Cells Translational Medicine. 2015;**4**(9):1033-1043

[33] Huh JW, Kim HR, Kim YJ, Lee JH, Park YS, Cho SH, et al. Expression of standard CD44 in human colorectal carcinoma: Association with prognosis. Pathology International. 2009;**59**:241-246

[34] Jing F, Kim HJ, Kim CH, Kim YJ, Lee JH, Kim HR. Colon cancer stem cell markers CD44 and CD133 in patients with colorectal cancer and synchronous hepatic metastases. International Journal of Oncology. 2015;**46**(4):1582-1588

[35] Ozawa M, Ichikawa Y, Zheng Y-W, Oshima T, Miyata H, Nakazawa K, et al. Prognostic significance of CD44 variant 2 upregulation in colorectal cancer. British Journal of Cancer. 2014;**111**:365-374

[36] Rohani P, Noroozinia F, Modarresi P, Abbasi A. CD44 standard isoform; not a good marker for colon cancer. International Journal of Cancer Management. 2017;**10**(9):e9166. DOI: 10.5812/ijcm.9166

[37] Matzke-Ogi A, Jannasch K, Shatirishvili M, Fuchs B, Chiblak S, Morton J, et al. Inhibition of tumor growth and metastasis in pancreatic cancer models by interference with CD44v6 signaling. Gastroenterology. 2016;**150**(2):513-525

[38] Zoller M. CD44: Can a cancer-initiating cell profit from an abundantly expressed molecule? Nature Reviews. Cancer. 2011;**11**:254-267

[39] Yeo M-K, Lee Y-M, Seong I-O, Choi S-Y, Suh K-S, Song KS, et al. Up-regulation of cytoplasmic CD24 expression is associated with malignant transformation but favorable prognosis of colorectal adenocarcinoma. Anticancer Research. 2016;**36**(12):6593-6598

[40] Weichert W, Denkert C, Burkhardt M, Gansukh T, Bellach J, et al. Cytoplasmic CD24 expression in colorectal cancer independently correlates with shortened patient survival. Clinical Cancer Research. 2005;**11**:6574-6581

[41] Marhaba R, Zoller M. CD44 in cancer progression: Adhesion, migration and growth regulation. Journal of Molecular Histology. 2004;**35**:211-231

[42] Du L, Wang H, He L, Zhang J, Ni B, et al. CD44 is of functional importance for colorectal cancer stem cells. Clinical Cancer Research. 2008;**14**:6751-6760

[43] Banky B, Raso-Barnett L, Barbai T, Timar J, Becsagh P, et al. Characteristics of CD44 alternative splice pattern in the course of human colorectal adenocarcinoma progression. Molecular Cancer. 2012;**11**:83

[44] Ahmed MA, Jackson D, Seth R, Robins A, Lobo DN, Tomlinson IP, et al. CD24 is upregulated in inflammatory bowel disease and stimulates cell motility and colony formation. Inflammatory Bowel Diseases. 2010;**16**:795-803

[45] Su N, Peng L, Xia B, Zhao Y, Xu A, Wang J, et al. Lyn is involved in CD24-induced ERK1/2 activation in colorectal cancer. Molecular Cancer. 2012;**11**

[46] Okano M, Konno M, Kano Y, Kim H, Kawamoto K, Ohkuma M, et al. Human colorectal CD24$^+$ cancer stem cells are susceptible to epithelia-mesenchymal transition. International Journal of Oncology. 2014;**45**:575-580

[47] Paschall AV, Yang D, Lu C, Redd PS, Choi J-H, Heaton CM, et al. CD133$^+$CD24^{lo} defines a 5-fluorouracil-resistant colon cancer stem cell-like phenotype. Oncotarget. 2016;**48**:78698-78712

[48] Seeber A, Untergasser G, Spizzo G, Terracciano L, Luigli A, Kasal A, et al. Predominant expression of truncated

EpCAM is associated with a more aggressive phenotype and predicts poor orverall survival in colorectal cancer. International Journal of Cancer. 2016;**139**(3):657-663

[49] Spizzo G, Fong D, Wurm M, Ensinger C, Obrist P, Hofer C, et al. EpCAM expression in primary tumor tissues and metastases: An immunohistochemical analysis. Journal of Clinical Pathology. 2011;**64**(5):415-420

[50] Zhou FQ , Qi YM, Xu H, Wang QY, Gao XS, Guo HG. Expresssion of EpCAM and Wnt/β-catenin in human colon cancer. Genetics and Molecular Research. 2015;**14**(2):4485-4494

[51] Wang A, Ramjeesingh R, Chen CH, Hurlbut D, Hammad N, Mulligan LM, et al. Reduction in membranous immunohistochemical staining for the intracellular domain of epithelial cell adhesion molecule correlates with poor patient outcome in primary colorectal adenocarcinoma. Current Oncology. 2016;**23**(3):e171-e178

[52] Manuel Simonab NS, Plückthunb A, Zangemeister-Wittke U. Epithelial cell adhesion molecule-targeted drug delivery for cancer therapy. Expert Opinion on Drug Delivery. 2013;**10**(4)

[53] Ulrike Schnell VC, Giepmans BN. EpCAM: Structure and function in health and disease. Biochimica et Biophysica Acta. 2013:1989-2001

[54] Yoon SM, Gerasimidou D, Kuwahara R, et al. Epithelial cell adhesion molecule (EpCAM) marks hepatocytes newly derived from stem/progenitor cells in humans. Hepatology. 2011;**53**(3):964-973

[55] Han S, Zong S, Hongijia L, Liu S, Yang W, Li W, et al. Is Ep-CAM expression a diagnostic and prognostic biomarker for colorectal cancer? A systematic meta-analysis. Cancers (Basel). 2017;**20**:61-69

[56] Vu T, Datta P. Regulation of EMT in colorectal cancer: A culprit in metastasis. Cancers (Basel). 2017;**9**(12):171

[57] Dolle L, Theise ND, Schmelzer E, et al. EpCAM and the biology of hepatic stem/progenitor cells. American Journal of Physiology. Gastrointestinal and Liver Physiology. 2015;**308**:G233-G250

[58] Mokhtari M, Zakerzade Z. EPCAM expression in colon adenocarcinoma and its relationship with TNM staging. Advanced Biomedical Research. 2017;**6**:56-63

[59] Joosse SA, Pantel K. Biologic challenges in the detection of circulating tumor cells. Cancer Research. 2013;**73**(1):8-11

[60] Wen L, Vivian CJ, Brinker AE, et al. Microenvironmental influences on metastasis suppressor expression and function during a metastatic cell's journey, 2014. Cancer Microenvironment. 2014;**7**:117-131

[61] Shafaei S, Sharbatdaran M, Kamrani G, Khafri S. The association between CD166 detection rate and clinicopathologic parameters of patients with colorectal cancer. Caspian Journal of Internal Medicine. 2013;**4**(4):768-772

[62] Hassan D, Vahid M, Ghanbar M, Habibollah M, Mohammad E, Nagres M. CD166 as a stem cell marker? A potential target for therapy colorectal cancer. Journal of Stem Cell Research & Therapeutics. 2016;**I**(6):226-229

[63] Ni C, Zhang Z, Zhu X, Liu Y, Qu D, Wu P, et al. Prognostic value of CD166 expression in cancers of the digestive system: A systematic review and meta-analysis. PloS one. 2013;**8**(8):e70958. DOI: 10.1371/journal.pone.0070958

[64] Weichert W, Knosel T, Bellach J, Dietel M, Kristiansen G. ALCAM/CD166 is overexpressed in

colorectal carcinoma and correlates with shortened patient survival. Journal of Clinical Pathology. 2004;**57**(11):1160-1164

[65] Tachezy M, Zander H, Gebauer F, Marx A, Kaifi JT, Izbicki JR, et al. Activated leukocyte cell adhesion molecule (CD166)—Its prognostic power for colorectal cancer patients. The Journal of Surgical Research. 2012;**177**(1):e15-e20

[66] Han S, Yang W, Zong S, Li H, Liu S, Li W, et al. Clinicopathological, prognostic and predictive value of CD166 expression in colorectal cancer: A meta-analysis. Oncotarget. 2017;**8**:64373-64384

[67] Levin TG, Powell AE, Davies PS, et al. Characterization of the intestinal cancer stem cell marker CD166 in the human and mouse gastrointestinal tract. Gastroenterology. 2010;**139**(6):2072-2082

[68] Hatano Y, Fukuda S, Hisamatsu K, Hirata A, Hara A, Tomita H. Multifacet interpretation of colon cancer stem cells. International Journal of Molecular Sciences. 2017;**18**(7):1446

[69] Fanali C, Luccetti D, Farina M, Corbi M, Cufino V, Cittadini A, et al. Cancer stem cells in colorectal cancer from pathogenesis to therapy: Controversies and perspectives. World Journal of Gastroenterology. 2014;**20**(4):923-942

[70] Wu XS, Xi HQ, Chen L. Lgr5 is a potential marker of colorectal carcinoma stem cells that correlates with patient survival. World Journal of Surgical Oncology. 2012;**10**:244

[71] Zheng Z, Yu H, Huang Q, Wu H, Fu Y, Shi J, et al. Heterogenous expression of Lgr5 as a risk factor for focal invasion and distant metastasis of colorectal carcinoma. Oncotarget. 2018;**9**(53):300025-300033

[72] Wahab R, Islam F, Gopalan V, Kin-yin LA. The identification and clinical implications of cancer stem cells in colorectal cancer. Clinical Colorectal Cancer. 2017;**16**(2):93-102

[73] Holah NS, Aiad HAES, Assad NY, Elkhouly EA, Lasheen AG. Evaluation of the role of ALDH1 as cancer stem cell marker in colorectal carcinoma: An immunohistochemical study. Journal of Clinical and Diagnostic Research. 2017;**11**(1):EC17-EC23

[74] Zhou F, Mu YD, Liang J, Liu ZX, Chen HS, Zhang JF. Expression and prognostic value of tumor stem cell markers ALDH1 and CD133 in colorectal carcinoma. Oncology Letters. 2014;**7**(2):507-512

[75] Mohamed SY, Kaf RM, Ahmed MM, Elwan A, Ashour HR, Ibrahim A. The prognostic value of cancer stem cell markers (Notch1, ALDH1, and CD44) in primary colorectal carcinoma. Journal of Gastrointestinal Cancer. 23 August 2018. DOI: 10.1007/s12029-018-0156-6. [Epub ahead of print]

[76] Chen J, Xia Q, Jiang B, Chang W, Yuan W, Ma Z, et al. Prognostic value of cancer stem cell marker ALDH1 expression in colorectal cancer: A systematic review and meta-analysis. PLoS One. 2015;**10**(12):e0145164

[77] Ueda K, Ogasawara S, Akiba J, Nakayama M, Todoroki K, Ueda K, et al. Aldehyde dehydrogenase 1 identifies cells with cancer stem cell-like properties in a human renal cell carcinoma cell line. PLoS One. 2013;**8**(10):e75463. DOI: 10.1371/journal.pone.0075463

[78] Goossens-Beumer I, Zeestraten E, Benard A, Christen T, Reimers M, Keijzer R, et al. The clinical prognostic value of combined analysis of Aldh1, Survivin, and EpCAM expression in colorectal cancer. British Journal of Cancer. 2014;**110**(12):2935-2944

Section 3

Clinical Surgery

Chapter 3

Laparoscopic Live Donor Nephrectomy: Techniques and Results

Maroun Moukarzel, Charbel Chalouhy, Nabil Harake and Freda Richa

Abstract

Living donation is still needed to overcome organ shortage. All countries seem to increase and encourage such kind of donation according to medical and ethical guidelines. The results of renal transplantation from living donors are better compared to those from cadaveric kidneys. Since the first successful kidney transplantation from a living donor, some 63 years ago, surgery has shifted toward a less invasive approach offering to the donor less pain, better cosmesis, a shorter hospital stay, and a quick return to normal activities. Laparoscopic living-donor nephrectomy (LLDN) is now considered as the gold standard approach for kidney retrieval on live donors and has undoubtedly revolutionized kidney donation. It must offer to the donor safety, low morbidity, and fast recovery and must obtain a graft with adequate vessel length, short warm ischemia time, and well-preserved ureteral blood supply. We describe our technique of LLDN according to safety principles and reproducible steps. Highly qualified and well-trained surgeons are allowed to perform such techniques within a very well-equipped environment and with experienced surgical staff. A living donor program should undertake at least 30 cases per year to maintain adequate experience and offer less complication rate.

Keywords: live donor, laparoscopy, nephrectomy, kidney transplantation, living kidney donation

1. Introduction

Living kidney donation has successfully improved the lives of many patients worldwide for over half a century. Do we still have the same need for living donors in 2018? The answer is obviously yes and for many reasons. The first is organ shortage with a widening gap between renal supply and demand in all countries that increases every year despite the use of marginal deceased donors. Waiting lists are growing everywhere. The site of the US Government Information on Organ Donation and Transplantation, organdonor.gov, shows recently a transplant waiting list of more than 114,000 patients of whom 83% are potential kidney recipients [1]. The second reason is the significant graft survival advantage and the reduction of the waiting time between end-stage renal disease and graft implantation. The results of renal transplantation from living donors are better compared to those from cadaveric kidneys with a graft half-life of 18 versus

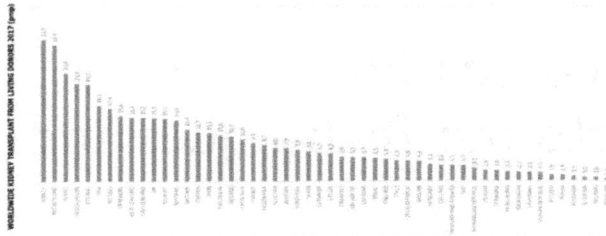

Figure 1.
Worldwide kidney transplant from living donors in 2017. International Registry in Organ Donation and Transplantation.

12 years, respectively [2]. Kidney transplantation from a living donor, when possible, is the best treatment for most patients with end-stage renal disease. This is related to multiple factors such as less time from dialysis to transplantation, shorter cold ischemia time, and better quality of the graft. The third reason stands for pediatric recipients where a prompt transplantation from a living donor, mostly a parent, can help for a better growth, quick return to school, and a good psychological stability; it is considered today as the gold standard therapy for children with end-stage renal disease. The fourth argument is that living donation provides a good opportunity to perform a preemptive transplantation avoiding the need of going through dialysis. A fifth reason is that we are still too far to overcome organ shortage by using xenografts from transgenic animals, or engineered organs from stem cells.

Currently, 40% of kidney grafts in the United States are from living donors [1]. In Europe, the level is highly variable between countries, standing for approximately 10% in France and up to 60% in Norway and Sweden [2, 3]. Approximately, one in three kidney transplants performed in the UK are from living donors [4], and according to the Global Observatory on Donation and Transplantation (GODT), 84,347 kidney transplants were done worldwide in 2015, of which 41.8% were from living donors [5].

In some countries, namely Middle Eastern and Eastern, kidney transplantation is relying only or mostly on living donors [6, 7]. Worldwide kidney transplant from living donors in 2017, based on the International Registry in Organ Donation and Transplantation, is shown in **Figure 1** [8].

Women traditionally outrank men in their enthusiasm to donate one of their kidneys. Although most recipients are male, women represented 63% of all living donations in 2016 [9].

In regard to these facts, living donors have exceptional courage and nobility; they go through a major surgery, accepting all surgical and medical risks and of no medical and physical benefit for them. It is our vocation and duty to provide them a safe and good practice according to legal and ethical bylaws and to protect their health in the long term.

2. Historical milestones

The first true altruistic voluntary living donation happened in Paris at Necker Hospital on December 25, 1952, when a mother, Gilberte Renard, convinced the medical team to give her kidney to her son Marius, 16 years old, apprentice carpenter who had his right solitary kidney removed after falling from a scaffolding. Unfortunately, the graft remained functional for approximately 3 weeks despite the use of steroids and Marius died on January 27, 1953. His donating mother died in 1992 at age 85 [10, 11].

The second important milestone happened 1 year later on December 23,1954 at Brigham Hospital in Boston USA, when Dr. Murray performed a successful renal transplantation on Richard Hersick, the donor being his monozygotic identical twin brother Ronald. The kidney was removed from Ronald by the urologist Harrison. No effort was made to preserve the isograft; but nonetheless, it functioned promptly despite 82 min of warm ischemia [12]. The graft remained functional for 8 years and was lost due to a recurrence of the renal disease and causing the death of Richard. His brother Ronald died in 2010 at age 79, after a cardiac surgery, just 4 days after the 56th anniversary of his pioneering kidney operation [11, 13].

The next two following years, the Brigham team performed seven successful kidney transplants also between identical twins. The most famous was that of Edith Helm, the third case at Brigham, who got pregnant 2 years after her transplant and was the first kidney recipient to carry to term and give birth to a child. Edith Helm also holds the record of the best graft longevity of 55 years; she died in 2011 at age 76, with a functioning graft. Her donating identical twin sister, Wanda Foster, gave birth three times following her kidney donation and was still alive in 2016 [11, 14].

In 1960, the first kidney transplantation between genetically nonrelated patients was performed using immunosuppression. Late in 1963, a conference near Washington DC was held to present the overall findings from 216 recipients of renal allografts. The results were not gratifying: 52% of all those receiving grafts from related donors had died, and 81% of those with kidneys from unrelated or cadaveric donors. Joseph Murray concluded at that time that "kidney transplantation is still highly experimental and not yet a therapeutic procedure." By 1965, 1 year survival rates of allografted kidneys from living related donors were much better approaching 80%, due to better immunosuppression [12, 15].

In 1987, Alexandre et al. in Belgium published a first series of ABO-incompatible (ABO-I) living donors using splenectomy and heavy immunosuppressive regimen in the recipient. Results were fairly optimal [16].

Then, since 1989 and due to organ shortage, most ABO-I kidney transplantations have taken place in Japan with recently published data showing an excellent long-term outcome. Currently, ABO-I reached approximately 30% of all living donor renal transplantation in Japan [17, 18].

From the surgical point of view, all donor nephrectomies were done by open techniques mostly using a lumbar retroperitoneal approach; and the first successful trial of removing a live donor kidney using a laparoscopic approach was in 1995 at John's Hopkins hospital by Ratner et al. [19]. Since then, considerable numbers of transplant centers worldwide have adopted laparoscopic donor nephrectomy (LDN) which is now considered as the gold standard approach for kidney retrieval on live donors and has undoubtedly revolutionized kidney donation.

3. Living donor evaluation

Suitability of the potential kidney recipient for transplantation must be established before starting donor assessment. There is a significant variability among transplant programs in the criteria used to evaluate donors. ABO blood grouping is an important early screening test. Initial assessment of donor and recipient histocompatibility status must be undertaken at an early stage in living donor kidney transplant workup to avoid unnecessary and invasive clinical investigation [4]. Although donors are not true patients, they must undergo a complete and extensive evaluation before considering kidney removal. This evaluation includes medical and surgical past history, risk factors like alcohol intake and smoking, family history (mainly renal disease, hypertension, and diabetes), renal, liver, and cardiopulmonary function. They should have no active malignancy or infection. The waiting period before transplant in recipients with a history of malignancy depends on the type, TNM stage and grade of the tumor, and recipient's age and general health. Recipients with tumors that have a low recurrence rate can be considered for immediate transplantation after successful treatment. Active HBV and HCV are usually contraindications to living donor kidney donation; and HIV infection is an absolute contraindication. Screening of serum prostate-specific antigen (PSA) is mandatory in males above 54 years as also mammograms in women. A urine albumin/creatinine ratio done on a spot urine sample is a recommended screening test and it should be <30 mg/mmol. The presence of persistent microhematuria (two or more positive urine analysis) or recently called "persistent nonvisible hematuria," with no evident explanation like stones, neoplasms, and infection, should be investigated with cystoscopy and renal biopsy. Assessment of renal function is based on serum creatinine and calculation of creatinine clearance. Differential kidney function, using DMSA isotope scanning, is recommended when there is >10% variation in kidney size or abnormal renal anatomy [4]. Donors with mild and well-controlled hypertension, on one or two antihypertensive drugs, and with no evidence of end organ damage (retinopathy, left ventricular hypertrophy, proteinuria), might be accepted [20]. Data regarding long-term safety of nephrectomy in hypertensive donors are modest; but small studies with short-term follow-up suggest no increase in the incidence of kidney disease or worsening of the control of hypertension in donors with a history of mild well-controlled hypertension [21]. The Amsterdam Forum consensus guidelines in 2004 stated that some patients (age > 50, GFR >80, and with low urine albumin excretion of <30 mg/d) with easily controlled hypertension can represent a low-risk group for the development of kidney disease but might be considered as donors [22]. A psychosocial assessment is recommended for all donors with appropriate referral to a mental health professional who can be a psychologist or a psychiatrist. This assessment also evaluates whether the decision to donate is free of constraint and other undue pressures. Donor age is suggested to be between 22 and 75 years; but the upper age limit can be beyond if the donor is in good health and with a normal range of age-related change in kidney function (e.g., advisory threshold GFR levels considered acceptable at age 80 years is 58 ml/min/1.73 m^2 for males and 49 ml/min/1.73 m^2 for females). A safe threshold level of predonation kidney function is one that leaves sufficient function after donation to maintain the donor in normal status without affecting lifespan [4]. Old donors (> 60 years) should be aware of a greater risk of pre- and postoperative complications. We are very cautious about young donors who are less than 30 years old because their absolute risk over a lifetime, particularly with additional risk factors for end-stage renal disease (like hypertension, obesity, and diabetes), is likely to be more significant [4]. Living donors should ideally have a body mass index (BMI) that is less than 30 kg/m^2. Data on the safety of kidney donation in the very obese (BMI >35 kg/m^2) are limited and donation should be discouraged. Morbid obesity increases the risk of hypertension, dyslipidemia, insulin resistance and diabetes, heart disease, stroke, sleep apnea, and certain cancers [23]. On the other hand, data suggest that laparoscopic living-donor nephrectomy (LLDN) is an increasingly safe procedure in the otherwise healthy obese kidney donor and does not result in a high rate of major perioperative complications [24, 25]. Also, transplantation from an old or obese donor is most probably better than dialysis or transplantation from a deceased donor [26]. Computed tomography and tomographic angiography are used to assess renal vascular anatomy (presence of accessory vessels, intervessel distance, distance from ostium to the first division, presence of atherosclerotic disease), renal dimensions, presence of stones, urinary tract anatomy, and the existence of any suspicious lesion not seen on ultrasound. Around 25% of will have multiple arteries to one kidney and 7% will have multiple vessels to both kidneys [27]. Renal pedicles with less than three arteries are accepted.

The presence of multiple renal cystic lesions in a potential living kidney donor requires careful evaluation and a detailed family history; in those with a family history of polycystic kidney disease under the age of 40 years, the presence of two or more cysts (unilateral or bilateral) indicates autosomal dominant polycystic disease (ADPKD) and exclude donation [28]. For those aged 40–59 years, the absence of at least two cysts in each kidney gives a 100% negative predictive value for ADPKD, while for those older, up to four cysts are acceptable in each kidney [4]. History or current presence of bilateral renal stones is a contra indication for donation; but in some centers, donors with a history of nephrolithiasis are accepted as long as stones are no longer present and metabolic studies are normal [29].

4. Surgical technique

Multiple techniques have been described to harvest a kidney from a living donor. The old classic open surgery performed through a lumbar or subcostal incision is nowadays much less popular compared to mini-invasive approaches using laparoscopic extra corporeal manipulation and magnified ultrahigh definition view of the surgical field. But regardless of how minimally invasive laparoscopy can be, living donor nephrectomy remains a maximally invasive surgery because we are dealing with major vessels and consequently very serious and sometimes lethal hemorrhagic complications might occur. Highly qualified, competent, and well-trained surgeons are allowed to perform such techniques within a very well-equipped environment and with experienced surgical staff. A living donor program should undertake at least 30 cases per year to maintain adequate experience. Today, laparoscopy is by far the preferred procedure for kidney removal in live donors, offering a quick recovery, less pain, and a shorter hospital stay; and it will be the technique detailed in this chapter. A well-informed consent is obtained prior to surgery. The surgeon performing living donor nephrectomy has a particular responsibility to ensure that the donor fully understands the potential risks and long-term effects of the operation. Surgery must offer to the donor safety, low morbidity, and fast recovery; and must obtain a graft with adequate vessel length, short warm ischemia time, and well-preserved ureteral blood supply. A donor kidney with a single renal artery should, whenever possible, be chosen for transplantation to minimize the risk of vascular complications in the recipient procedure; similarly, single renal veins are usually preferred. Many transplant centers prefer the left kidney for LLDN because of the longer vein and perhaps an easier surgery on the left side; but with increasing experience, kidney side was not a real obstacle [30] although for some authors the right kidney was the only risk factor for early graft thrombosis [31, 32]. The answer to which kidney to take when facing a donor with two arteries on the left and a single artery on the right is based on the surgeon's experience of laparoscopic right nephrectomy and his skills in reconstructing the vasculature of the graft. The presence of a retroaortic renal vein is of no problem with no increased complications; and it is even an easier case because of the large distance between the artery and the retroaortic vein which is in an inferior position (**Figure 2**). The most important criterion regarding the side to be chosen for retrieval is to keep the better kidney for the living donor.

There is variability among different centers on the choice of laparoscopic technique between only pure laparoscopy (transperitoneal versus retroperitoneal), only hand-assisted laparoscopy or a combination of both. Laparoendoscopic single-site

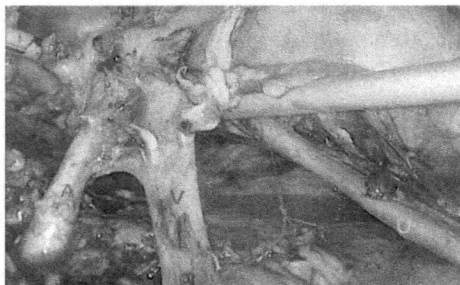

Figure 2.
Retroaortic vein (V). See the distance between the artery (A) and the vein (V). U = ureter.

surgery (LESS), natural orifice transluminal endoscopic surgery (NOTES), and robotic-assisted are other interesting techniques that still need to be evaluated. In our experience, we started our first 10 cases with hand assistance, given the increased security that it provides, and then switched to pure transperitoneal laparoscopic approach which will be detailed in this chapter.

4.1 Anesthesia

Laparoscopic donor nephrectomy has had a big impact on anesthesia and recovery of this special category of patients. Intraoperative anesthesia for laparoscopic live donors follows the rules of laparoscopic kidney surgery as far as sedation and muscle relaxation but the concept of protection of the donor kidney is mandatory throughout the case, one among many disparities compared to other kidney surgeries [33]. Nowadays, two large-bore IV catheters are considered more than enough as far as vascular access and risk of bleeding. Arterial lines are not recommended and noninvasive blood pressure monitoring is a reasonable option [34]. After induction of anesthesia, classically with propofol and a neuromuscular blocking agent, maintenance of anesthesia has been the subject of many studies to evaluate the nephrotoxicity of various agents. While isoflurane and desflurane were considered safe and with the least toxicity on the kidney, this was not the case with sevoflurane that is associated with production of compound A in the circulation; a direct nephrotoxic substance [35]. Despite many works, the type of anesthetic agent was not shown to impact serum creatinine or GFR in transplanted grafts and it was concluded that toxicity, if any, was minimal. Nitrous oxide is one agent preferably avoided in laparoscopic surgery as it can cause bowel distention in more than 50% of cases and subsequent compromise of insufflation or surgical field exposure in near 25% of laparoscopic donor nephrectomy, increasing the need even more for neuromuscular blocking agents [36]. Mechanical ventilation settings are not different from other laparoscopic procedures. Special considerations for donor nephrectomy would include tolerance of mild hypercapnia to 45 mmHg since it helps better tissue perfusion and circulation in light of pneumoperitoneum. Positive-end expiratory pressure (PEEP) at 5–10 mmHg, a 20–30% increase in minute ventilation reflecting an increased respiratory rate with constant volumes, is similar to other laparoscopic procedures. The effects of pneumoperitoneum were explored by studies on rats demonstrating that abdominal insufflation with CO_2 during laparoscopy in subjects with chronic renal function impairment should not be a contraindication to surgery [37]. Additionally, if insufflation had a substantial negative effect on kidney function, we would have expected this to have a great impact on kidney donors out of concern on the retained kidney, which has not been born out in the literature. IV hydration holds a crucial place in counteracting the notorious effects of pneumoperitoneum on tissue perfusion and renal plasma flow caused by an increased intraperitoneal pressure sometimes near 15 mmHg. Some studies emphasized the great effects of hydration on mean arterial pressure preservation and ensuring hemodynamic stability [38]. Whether this is realized by giving donors colloid boluses preoperatively or during surgery is based on institutional protocols and the team preferences. In general, a patient undergoing laparoscopic donor nephrectomy should get 4–6 L during the procedure to maintain at least a urine output >50 mL/h [38]. This will help avoid the use of any vasopressors or inotrope agents because of the associated deleterious renal vasoconstriction. If they become really needed, ephedrine is the best agent to start with, giving small boluses in order to attain the desired effects. IV fluids should be warmed and full measures should be taken to prevent hypothermia. There is a mounting evidence to suggest that 0.9% normal saline can be detrimental to patient outcome, and may indeed contribute to renal dysfunction, and therefore, the use of this solution in donors cannot be recommended; Ringer's lactate solution is the intravenous fluid of choice [4]. The administration of mannitol 12–25 g once or twice, or furosemide at small doses during the case, is another example of common practice depending on departmental protocols, but they lack any definite data or evidence to support it.

4.2 Antibiotics, patient position, and trocar placement

We routinely give antibiotic prophylaxis based on one single shot of cefazolin. After placement of a Foley catheter, the patient is put in a complete lateral decubitus position almost 90° to the table without any flexure or kidney rest; the belly being on the external border of the table. Arms and legs are well secured with pillows and gel pads to prevent any vascular or nerve compression. We start by doing the extraction site as a small transverse supra pubic incision 6–8 cm width, depending on donor kidney size, with opening of the peritoneum and insertion of a LapCap device (Applied Medical-Alexis Laparoscopic System with Kii® Fios® First Entry) (**Figure 3** and Video 1 (https://youtu.be/LBWXDCD2Upk)). Pneumoperitoneum induction is made through this device. Intraabdominal CO_2 pressure is fixed at 12 mm Hg. The use of low-pressure pneumoperitoneum with deep neuromuscular block did not seem to reduce postoperative pain scores or improve the overall quality of recovery after surgery [39]. After complete insufflation, we insert all trocars under direct vision. On the left side, the first is a 10 mm placed umbilical or para umbilical depending on obesity status; the second is a 5 mm placed subcostal on the level of the anterior axillary line, and the third one is a 12 mm trocar (which comes in the LapCap package) placed in the left iliac fossa (**Figure 3**). On the right side,

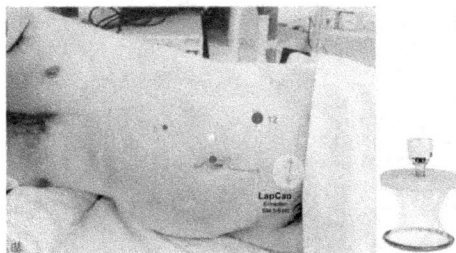

Figure 3.
Left side: position of patient and 3 trocar placement: 5 mm subcostal, 10 mm umbilical or para umbilical (yellow dot) depending on obesity, and 12 mm left iliac fossa. LapCap device shown on the right.

trocar placement is the same with an additional 5 mm one, inserted at the xiphoid for liver retraction. Additional ports can be used in some rare difficult cases and sometimes we do percutaneous kidney suspension using a 2/0 silk on a straight needle through Gerota's fascia and perirenal fat (**Figure 4**).

4.3 Surgical steps

As described in all transperitoneal approaches, we start by taking the colon off the kidney medially along the Toldt's fascia from the iliac vessels up to the colonic angle (splenic flexure on the left and hepatic flexure on the right). Gerota's fascia is left intact on the kidney (**Figure 5**). The lateral and parietal attachments of the kidney are left in place to prevent the kidney from slipping down and disturbing later the hilar dissection. We use from the start a LigaSure™ Maryland 5 mm (Covidien) sealing device. We then dissect and isolate the ureter inferiorly down to the iliac vessels with identification of the psoas muscle and the genital vessels. All periureteral and inferior renal pole fat must be well preserved to keep a well-vascularized ureter (**Figure 6**). Avoid any injury to the genitofemoral nerve and try to keep the psoas fascia in place. The gonadal vein can be divided proximally and distally and kept with the ureter in order to protect ureteric vascularity. This is thought to be the cause of postoperative ipsilateral orchialgia, which occurs in 6.2–9.6% of male donors [40, 41]. Large studies, however, have demonstrated that leaving the gonadal vein in situ does not lead to increased ureteric complications in the transplant recipient [42] and prevents orchialgia [40, 43].

4.3.1 Left-sided nephrectomy

The ureter and its peri ureteral fat are lifted up to undertake an upper dissection along the genital vein until we reach the inferior border and the anterior aspect of the renal vein (Video 2 (https://youtu.be/Ms38M9mIV0Q)). Then, the spleen and tail of the pancreas are completely mobilized by cutting the splenorenal and splenophrenic ligaments (Video 3 (https://youtu.be/lKNHPx66Mgo)). Care is taken not to injure the pancreas, the splenic artery, and the stomach near the level of the crus of the diaphragm where dissection ends. By achieving this step, the space between the spleen and the kidney is usually widely opened and permits partial mobilization of the upper renal pole (**Figure 7**). We then proceed to adrenal dissection and separation starting very carefully from the upper border of the renal vein toward the upper pole of the kidney with division of the adrenal vein using LigaSure sealing without any clip placement and caring not to injure the anterior branch of the renal artery or small upper pole accessory

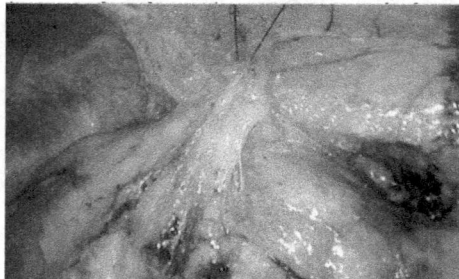

Figure 4.
Left kidney suspended with a 2/0 silk suture on the parietal wall.

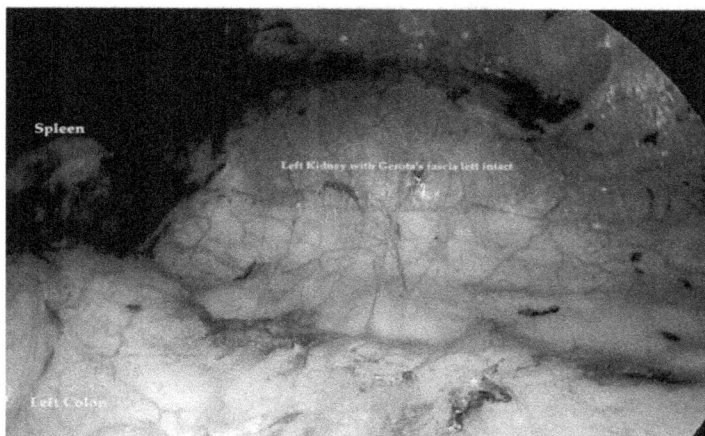

Figure 5.
Left renal aspect after colon dissection. Gerota's fascia is left intact.

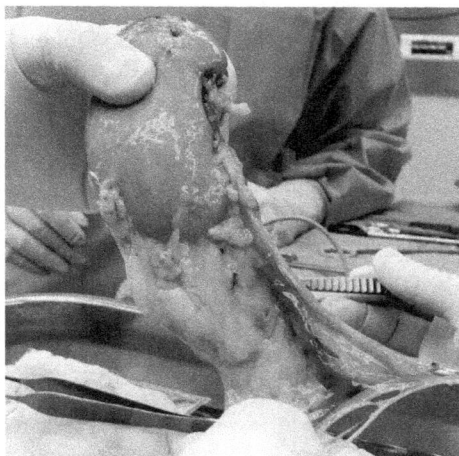

Figure 6.
Ureter with well-preserved periureteral fat and vasculature.

arteries not detected on the preoperative renal angio CT scan (Video 4 (https://youtu. be/WbgzAzZZprk)). This step will almost complete the upper pole release.

The renal pedicle is now ready to be dissected. Before starting the hilar dissection, 12–25 mg of mannitol is administered. All lymphatics and autonomic nerve plexuses superior to the vein and around the renal artery are sealed and cut. Some small segments of these structures are sometimes difficult or possibly dangerous to access, and in such a case, they are quickly sealed and cut after the stapling of the renal pedicle. Very careful and minutious dissection is undertaken between the artery and vein to prepare a clear, precise, and secure positioning of the stapling device. The left renal artery is dissected at its aortic origin (Video 5 (https:// youtu.be/5wyqkJz7ick)). If vasospasm is noted, the renal artery can be bathed in a papaverine solution (30 mg/ml) [44]. In some cases, retroperitoneal veins (lumbar, ascending lumbar, and hemiazygos) join the left renal vein in up to 75% of individuals, and it must be sealed and cut [45]. Clips are avoided on all venous branches

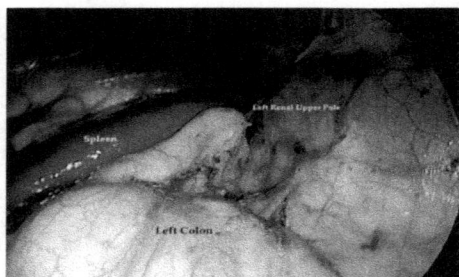

Figure 7.
Spleen separated from the left renal upper pole.

to prevent their later insertion between the jaws of the stapling device leading to misfire and serious malfunction [46].

The ureter and its periureteral fat are again lifted up at the level of the iliac vessels and posterior dissection will start from here and go up to the whole posterior surface of the kidney. The ureter is isolated with a generous periureteric fat. After completing this posterior release, the kidney is completely lying medially and we can free the posterior aspect of the renal artery (**Figure 8**; Video 6 (https://youtu. be/xQswiMds4Nc)). Now the kidney is supposed to hold only on the artery, vein, and ureter and is ready to be harvested. The patient is given another dose of mannitol. An Endocatch bag 15 mm (Covidien) is inserted through the LapCap. The distal ureter is clipped and sectioned. A good flow of urine should be noticed before pedicle clamping. A number of vascular transfixing stapling devices are available for surgeons to secure the renal vessels. The choice of which device to use is down to surgeon preference. Recently, we rely on two stapling devices: Endo-TA 30 stapler (30-mm length, 2.5-mm staples-Covidien) if maximum length is needed because this device delivers three rows of staplers without a cutting knife and no articulation; and vessels are cut with cold scissors; and Echelon Flex™ Powered Vascular Stapler 35 mm (Ethicon) with manual articulation for more precise placement, a narrow curved blunt tip, and reduction in tip movement during firing; this device delivers four rows of staples (instead of six) in a staggered pattern and gives a very secure vascular control and less loss in vessel length with nonbloody surgical field because of the absent backflow. Stapling starts on the renal artery and then quickly on the vein, and the kidney is rapidly placed in the Endo bag and extracted through the LapCap (Videos 7 (https://youtu.be/RfIGOjtqpD8) and 8 (https://youtu.be/ dGUKd3R23Yo)). We do not give intravenous heparin prior to vascular occlusion.

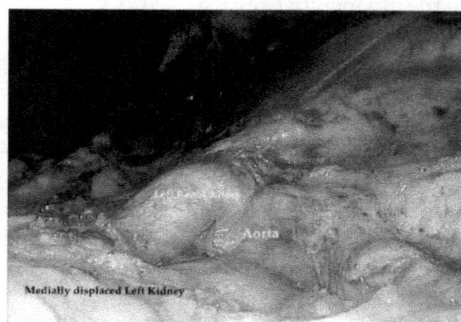

Figure 8.
Laparoscopic view after posterior left renal dissection.

Warm ischemia time is usually around 3–5 min before the kidney is flushed out on ice with the preservation solution.

Originally, the artery was secured using locking polymer clips that are much cheaper than staples. On April 2006, the manufacturer of Weck Hem-o-lok ligating clips, Teleflex Medical, added a contraindication to the use of these clips on renal vessels in laparoscopic live donor nephrectomy, after receiving 15 medical device reports of 12 injuries and 3 deaths, all of which occurred between November 19, 2001 and March 20, 2005. All reports were associated with using the clips for ligation of the renal artery during LLDN [47, 48]. Clip dislodgement may occur several hours following the procedure resulting in fatal hemorrhage on the ward [49]. US Food and Drug Administration (FDA) issued on May 2011 a warning to healthcare providers that Weck Hem-o-Lok ligating clips should not be used for the ligation of the renal artery during LLDN because of serious risks and potential life-threatening complications to the donor [50]. On the other hand, surgeons must be aware that reported failure rates for staplers are 3.0% [51]. Stapler misfire rates can be reduced by avoiding the use of titanium and other clips around the hilar structures before securing the renal pedicle [46].

Before ending the surgery, latero aortic and inter aorto caval lymphatics are clipped (Hem-o-lok clips) to prevent chylous leakage (Video 9 (https://youtu.be/_c4rjTtvlTw)). Meticulous and extensive clipping remains the safest way of securing lymphatic channels along the dissection area despite being usually burned with energy-based sealing devices. It has been shown that bipolar cautery can effectively ligate and control lymph leakage as also other laparoscopic dissection devices using bipolar and ultrasonic energy but monopolar scissors were unreliable with respect to sealing lymphatic channels [52, 53]. Last view of the whole surgical field is done with particular inspection of the vascular stumps (**Figure 9**). Pneumoperitoneum is exsufflated. No drainage is usually needed. Port and extraction sites are closed.

4.3.2 Right-sided nephrectomy

In some patients, the right side seems to be easier than the left. Steps are almost the same. Trocar placement has the same distribution as on the left except for an additional 5 mm trocar inserted at the xiphoid for liver retraction (**Figure 10**). Less right colon dissection is needed and careful duodenal displacement is performed to expose the inferior vena cava (IVC). Genital vein is usually kept in place. The renal upper pole is carefully separated from the adrenal as on the left side starting from the upper border of the right vein. Renal vessels are also approached from below after isolation of the ureter and periureteral fat and identification of the psoas muscle and lifting up the kidney. The right renal vein is exposed at its insertion into

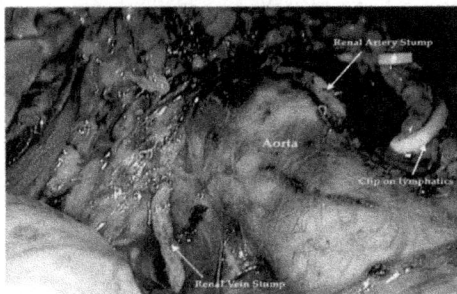

Figure 9.
Left renal artery and vein stumps after stapling and kidney harvesting. Clips on lymphatics are placed after vascular stapling.

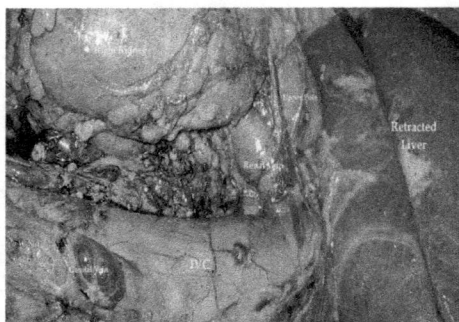

Figure 10.
Liver retracted through a 5-mm xiphoid trocar.

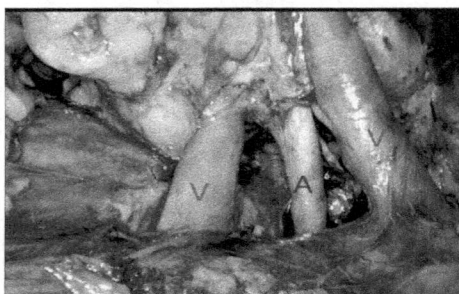

Figure 11.
Laparoscopic view of right donor kidney with two veins (V) and one artery (A).

the IVC. Duplication of renal vein is more common on the right side and is reported in as much as 15% of potential renal donors [54] (**Figure 11**). The adrenal vein, gonadal vein, and retroperitoneal veins (lumbar, ascending lumbar, and hemiazygos) may drain into the right renal vein in 30, 7, and 3% of cases, respectively [55]. The IVC must be well dissected below and above the renal vein to permit later easy positioning of the stapler device. In usual anatomy, the renal artery is classically found just behind the vein and the space between artery and vein is normally easily created. Retrocaval area is a difficult area to work at during LLDN; therefore, the exact location of the first segmental branch of right renal artery with respect to the IVC should be clearly identified in the pretransplant angio CT scan. In some cases, posterior release of the artery behind the IVC is necessary to reach the main trunk (Video 10 (https://youtu.be/DPGFtpAVar8)) especially if the artery is in an upper position to the vein (Video 11 (https://youtu.be/BfbPdO-U8zU)); or even rarely, access to the artery is done through the inter aorto caval space. Caval countertraction is applied just prior to firing the endovascular stapler, so that adequate venous length is obtained. The renal vein is usually 2–3 mm shorter compared with the open surgery. Operative time and warm ischemia time may be greater when performing a right-sided LLDN, but this does not result in delayed allograft function [56].

5. Postoperative care

The early postoperative period after laparoscopic donor nephrectomy is a particular moment in the management of kidney donors. Extubation is done after normothermic state. Orogastric tube is removed prior to extubation. Hemoglobin measurement is realized every 6 h postsurgery, and if normal, it will be repeated the next morning with serum creatinine and electrolytes. Urine output is monitored. Shoulder tip discomfort and pain is a major complaint after LLDN perhaps from residual pneumoperitoneum. Epidural analgesia is ineffective for shoulder pain. There has been collective belief to aggressively minimize pain postoperatively in this special category of patients who are usually narcotics naïve. IV "patient-controlled analgesia" (PCA; fentanyl or morphine less commonly) was considered to be the modality of choice to achieve that. If PCA is not available, pain control is achieved with IV paracetamol and if needed ketoprofen or ketorolac over the first 24 h [57]. To reduce the risk of nephrotoxicity, the patient should be kept well hydrated. Opiates also have an effective role for breakthrough pain when opiate-sparing strategies have not been effective. Clear liquids are started on the day of surgery with increase of diet later. The emergence of enhanced recovery after surgery (ERAS) brought major changes to the traditional standard of care. Many centers across the USA have adopted the enhanced recovery programs that include intraoperative fluid restriction to 3 ml/kg/h preventing excessive third spacing and bowel edema, urine output of 0.5 ml/kg/h, use of local subfascial bupivacaine or other anesthetics as well as a postoperative narcotic-free pain control regimen, i.e., acetaminophen, ketorolac, etc. [58]. Novelties in this management were associated with reduced length of hospital stay, better pain control, and increased patient satisfaction. It has become evident that ERAS would potentially enhance the benefits of laparoscopic surgery for kidney donors [59].

Foley catheter is removed on the morning of day 1 and ambulation started as soon as possible either during the evening of day 0 or the next morning. Living kidney donors are classified as "medium risk" patients for deep venous thrombosis (DVT) and pulmonary embolism [4]. All living donors must have intra- and post-operative compression stockings and should receive adequate thromboprophylaxis with low-molecular weight-heparin and continuing for at least 1 week. Patient is discharged most frequently on day 2 and seen back 10 days later with a follow-up at 6 months, 1 year, and 2 years after donation. Donors must resume a normal life-style as soon as possible with regular surveillance of their blood pressure and their weight. They should be warned about avoiding nephrotoxic medications.

6. Complications

LLDN appears to be a safe procedure or at least as safe as the open one. But serious complications including death may occur. Overall mortality rate is approximately 0.03% [34] although some large series reported no mortality [60–63]. Most of these deaths occurred in the postoperative period and were due to hemorrhage [47], CO_2 gas embolism [64], and pulmonary embolism [34]. The risk of a major intraoperative hemorrhage during LLDN is between 0.6 and 1.6% [60, 63]. Conversion to open surgery has been reported to occur in 0 to 13% of cases, but in most large series, conversion rates of 1–2% are reported [4, 60–63]. Other intraoperative complications are splenic or liver laceration, ureteral and intestinal injury, and pleural laceration. The total incidence of surgical complications is 5.46% [61]. All major complications occurred in the first 100 cases [62]. This raises the question of the learning curve and how many laparoscopic nephrectomies should be done before performing the first LLDN? There is no precise answer but a number between 50 and 100 seems to be convincing for this type of surgery to be learned.

Postoperative complications of LLDN are hematomas, fever, urinary tract infection, pneumonia, pulmonary embolism, wound infection, incisional hernias, prolonged ileus, chylous ascites, and left testicular pain perhaps due to gonadal vein division or extensive mobilization of the left colon which may damage the neural plexus supplying the testis and may also disrupt lymphatic drainage [65]. Chylous leakage is a rare complication of LLDN. Prevention is assured by doing a meticulous and extensive clipping of lymphatic channels along the dissection area [52, 66].

Long-term complications are arterial hypertension, renal failure, and proteinuria, particularly in more high-risk donors, such as those with obesity, old or young donors, hypertensive donors, and those with kidney stones [67, 68]. Following kidney donation, there is a compensatory increase in function in the remaining kidney. By 3 months, remnant kidney clearance increases to a mean GFR of around 65–75% of predonation renal function [4]. The average decrease in GFR after donation was 26 mL/min/1.73 m^2 (range 8–50) [4, 69]. The incidence of end-stage renal disease (ESRD) in living kidney donors appears to be similar to or lower than that seen in the unselected general population despite a reduction in GFR [4, 24, 70]. The estimated lifetime risk of ESRD was 90 per 10,000 in donors, 326 per 10,000 in the general population, and 14 per 10,000 in matched healthy nondonor controls [71]. Live donor nephrectomy alone will not lead to renal failure [72].

Concerning hypertension, a large meta-analysis demonstrated that donors have an increased systolic blood pressure of 5 mmHg after 5–10 years from donation [73]. The rate of hypertension in donors was similar to that of the general population [74]. But it seems that there are no effects on kidney function and microalbuminuria at least in Caucasian population. Blacks and Hispanics may have higher risks of hypertension-associated kidney disease after donation [75, 76].

Finally, it is interesting to know that longevity of live donors remains greater compared to the general population [24, 72, 77].

7. Conclusion

Living donation is a success story that saved many patients with end-stage renal disease from dialysis and offered them a better quality of life and longer life expectancy. Donor surgery has shifted from the old open technique to a mini-invasive approach that offers less pain to this category of people who are not true patients but true heroes full of courage and nobility. Ensuring the safety and excellent long-term outcomes of these donors is our duty, through all steps from preoperative workup, surgery, and postoperative care.

Donors must be aware of all potential complications before acceptance and should feel free to resign at any moment. Complications of LLDN are present and must be prevented by entrusting them to highly qualified and experienced surgeons.

Author details

Maroun Moukarzel[1*], Charbel Chalouhy[1], Nabil Harake[1] and Freda Richa[2]

1 Division of Urology and Kidney Transplantation, Hôtel Dieu de France University Hospital, Saint Joseph University Medical School, Beirut, Lebanon

2 Anesthesia and Intensive Care Department, Hôtel Dieu de France University Hospital, Saint Joseph University Medical School, Beirut, Lebanon

*Address all correspondence to: marounmoukarzel@gmail.com

IntechOpen

References

[1] US Government Information on Organ Donation and Transplantation. Available from: https://organdonor.gov [Accessed: 24 June, 2018]

[2] Delaporte V. Transplantation rénale à partir d'un donneur vivant. Progrès en Urologie. 2011;**21**:789-792. DOI: 10.1016/j.purbl.2011.09.003

[3] Hiesse C. Kidney transplantation epidemiology in France. Néphrologie & Thérapeutique. 2013;**9**(6):441-450. DOI: 10.1016/j. nepho.2013.02.002

[4] Guidelines for Living Donor Kidney Transplantation. Fourth Edition: March 2018. British Transplantation Society and The Renal Association. BTS/RA. http://www.bts.org.uk

[5] Global Observatory on Donation and Transplantation. Available from: http://www.transplant-observatory.org/Pages/Home.aspx [Accessed: 24 June, 2018]

[6] Ali A, Hendawy A. Renal transplantation in the Middle East: Strengths, weaknesses, opportunities and threats (SWOT) analysis. Urology & Nephrology Open Access Journal. 2015;**2**(2):00028. DOI: 10.15406/unoaj.2015.02.00028

[7] Shaheen FA, Souqiyyeh MZ. Current obstacles to organ transplant in Middle Eastern countries. Experimental and Clinical Transplantation. 2015;**13**(Suppl 1):1-3. PMID: 25894118

[8] International Registry in Organ Donation and Transplantation. Available from: http://www.irodat.org/?p=database [Accessed: 27 June, 2018]

[9] Gill J, Joffres Y, Rose C, Lesage J, Landsberg D, Kadatz M, et al. The change in living kidney donation in women and men in the United States (2005-2015): A population-based analysis. Journal of the American

Society of Nephrology. 2018;**29**:1301-1308; published ahead of print March 8, 2018. DOI: 10.1681/ASN.2017111160

[10] Michon L, Hamburger J, Oeconomos N, Delinotte P, Richet G, Vaysse J, et al. An attempted kidney transplantation in man: Medical and biological aspects. Presse Médicale. 1953;**61**:1419-1423

[11] Timsit MO, Kleinclauss F, Thuret R. History of kidney transplantation surgery. Progrès en Urologie. 2016;**26**:874-881. DOI: 10.1016/j.parol.2016.08.003

[12] History of Renal Transplant—Renal Medicine. Available from: www.renalmed.co.uk/history-of/renal-transplant [Accessed: 27 June, 2018]

[13] Merrill JP, Murray JE, Harrison J, Guild W. Successful homotransplantation of the human kidney between identical twins. Journal of the American Medical Association. 1956;**160**(4):277-282. PMID: 13278189

[14] Murray JE. Edith Helm (April 29, 1935–April 4, 2011): The world's longest surviving transplant recipient: Letter to the editor. American Journal of Transplantation. 2011;**11**:1545-1546. DOI: 10.1111/j.1600-6143.2011.03607.x

[15] Joseph E Murray. Nobel Prize Lecture: The first successful transplants in man. Presented on 8 December 1990, at Karolinska Institutet, Stockholm

[16] Squifflet J-P, De Meyer M, Malaise J, Latinne D, Pirson Y, Alexandre GPJ. Lessons learned from ABO-incompatible living donor kidney transplantation: 20 years later. Experimental and Clinical Transplantation. 2004;**2**(1):208-213. PMID: 15859930

[17] Takahashi K, Saito K, Takahara S, Okuyama A, Tanabe K, Toma H,

et al. Excellent long-term outcome
of ABO-incompatible living donor
kidney transplantation in Japan.
American Journal of Transplantation.
2004;**4**(7):1089-1096. PMID: 15196066.
DOI: 10.1111/j.1600-6143.2004.00464.x

[18] Tai Yeon Koo, Jaeseok Yang.
Current progress in ABO-incompatible
kidney transplantation; open access
article under the CC BY-NC-ND
license (http://creativecommons.org/
licenses/by-nc-nd/4.0/). DOI 10.1016/j.
krcp.2015.08.005

[19] Ratner LE, Ciseck LJ, Moore RG,
Cigarroa FG, Kaufman HS, Kavoussi
LR. Laparoscopic live donor
nephrectomy. Transplantation.
1995;**60**(9):1047-1049. [MEDLINE:
7491680]

[20] Karpinski M, Knoll G, Cohn A,
et al. The impact of accepting living
kidney donors with mild hypertension
or proteinuria on transplantation rates.
American Journal of Kidney Diseases.
2006;**47**:317-323

[21] Towsend RR, Reese PP, Lim
MA. Should living kidney donors
with hypertension be considered for
organ donation? Current Opinion
in Nephrology and Hypertension.
2015;**24**(6):594-601. DOI: 10.1097/
MNH.0000000000000169

[22] Delmonico F. A report of the
Amsterdam Forum on the care of the
live kidney donor: Data and medical
guidelines. Transplantation. 2005;**79**:S53

[23] Nguyen NT, Magno CP, Lane KT,
Hinojosa MW, Lane JS. Association of
hypertension, diabetes, dyslipidemia,
and metabolic syndrome with obesity:
Findings from the national health and
nutrition examination survey, 1999 to
2004. Journal of the American College
of Surgeons. 2008;**207**:928-934

[24] Segev DL, Muzaale AD, Caffo BS,
et al. Perioperative mortality and

long-term survival following live kidney
donation. Journal of the American
Medical Association. 2010;**303**:959-966

[25] Lentine KL, Lam NN, Axelrod
D, et al. Perioperative complications
after living kidney donation: A
national study. American Journal of
Transplantation. 2016;**16**:1848-1857

[26] Johnson SR et al. Older living donors
provide excellent quality kidneys: A
single center experience (older living
donors). Clinical Transplantation.
2005;**19**(5):600-606

[27] Weinstein SH, Navarre RJ, Loening
SA, Corry RJ. Experiences with live
donor nephrectomy. The Journal of
Urology. 1980;**124**:321-323

[28] Pei Y, Obaji J, Dupuis A, et al.
Unified criteria for ultrasonographic
diagnosis of ADPKD. Journal of the
American Society of Nephrology.
2009;**20**:205-212

[29] Mandelbrot DA, Pavlakis M,
Danovitch GM, Johnson SR, Karp SJ,
Khwaja K, et al. The medical evaluation
of living kidney donors: A survey of US
transplant centers. American Journal of
Transplantation. 2007;**7**(10):2333-2343.
[PubMed: 17845567]

[30] Liu N et al. Maximizing the donor
pool: Left versus right laparoscopic
live donor nephrectomy—Systematic
review and meta-analysis.
International Urology and Nephrology.
2014;**46**(8):1511. DOI: 10.1007/
s11255-014-0671-8. Epub Mar 5,
2014. https://www.ncbi.nlm.nih.gov/
pubmed/24595603

[31] Amézquita Y, Mendez C, Fernandez
A, et al. Risk factors for early renal
graft thrombosis: A case controlled
study in grafts from the same donor.
Transplantation Proceedings.
2008;**40**(9):2891-2893. DOI: 10.1016/j.
transproceed.2008.09.014

[32] Hsu JW, Reese PP, Naji A, Levine MH, Abt PL. Increased early graft failure in right-sided living donor nephrectomy. Transplantation. 2011;**91**(1):108-114. DOI: 10.1097/TP.0b013e3181fd0179

[33] Joshi GP, Cunningham A. Anesthesia for laparoscopic and robotic surgeries. In: Barash PG, editor. Clinical Anesthesia. Vol. 7th. Philadelphia: Lippincott Williams Wilkins; 2013. pp. 1257-1273

[34] Matas AJ, Bartlett ST, Leichtman AB, Delmonico FL. Morbidity and mortality after living kidney donation, 1999-2001: Survey of United States transplant centers. American Journal of Transplantation. 2003;**3**:830

[35] Ong Sio LCL, Dela Cruz RGC, et al. A comparison of renal responses to sevoflurane and isoflurane in patients undergoing donor nephrectomy: A randomized controlled trial. Medical Gas Research. 2017;**7**(1):19-27. eCollection 2017 Jan–Mar

[36] El-Galley R, Hammontree L, et al. Anesthesia for laparoscopic donor nephrectomy: Is nitrous oxide contraindicated? The Journal of Urology. 2007;**178**(1):225-227

[37] Dolkart O et al. Pneumoperitoneum in the presence of acute and chronic kidney injury: An experimental model in rats. The Journal of Urology. 2014;**192**:1266-1271. DOI: 10.1016/j.juro.2014.03.114

[38] Mertens zur Borg IRA, Di Biase M, Verbrugge S, IJzermans JNM, Gommers D. Comparison of three perioperative fluid regimes for laparoscopic donor nephrectomy: A prospective randomized dose-finding study. Surgical Endoscopy. 2008;**22**(1):146-150. Published online 24 May, 2007. PMCID: PMC2169269; PMID: 17522928. DOI: 10.1007/s00464-007-9391-9

[39] Brunschot D O-v, Scheffer GJ, van der Jagt M, Langenhuijsen H, Dahan A, Mulder JEEA, et al. Quality of recovery after low-pressure laparoscopic donor nephrectomy facilitated by deep neuromuscular blockade: A randomized controlled study. World Journal of Surgery. 2017;**41**:2950-2958. DOI: 10.1007/s00268-017-4080-x

[40] Shirodkar SP, Gorin MA, Sageshima J, et al. Technical modification for laparoscopic donor nephrectomy to minimize testicular pain: A complication with significant morbidity. American Journal of Transplantation. 2011;**11**:1031-1034

[41] Kim FJ, Pinto P, Su LM, et al. Ipsilateral orchialgia after laparoscopic donor nephrectomy. Journal of Endourology. 2003;**17**:405-409

[42] Kocak B, Baker TB, Koffron AJ, Leventhal JR. Ureteral complications in the era of laparoscopic living donor nephrectomy: Do we need to preserve the gonadal vein with the specimen? Journal of Endourology. 2010;**24**:247-251

[43] Banga N, Nicol D. Techniques in laparoscopic donor nephrectomy. BJU International. 2012;**110**:1368-1373. DOI: 10.1111/j.1464-410X.2012.11058.x

[44] Simforoosh N, Bassiri A, Ziaee SA, Maghsoodi R, Salim NS, Shafi H, et al. Laparoscopic versus open live donor nephrectomy: The first randomized clinical trial. Transplantation Proceedings. 2003;**35**:2553-2554

[45] Arévalo Pérez J, Gragera Torres F, Marín Toribio A, et al. Angio CT assessment of anatomical variants in renal vasculature: Its importance in the living donor. Insights into Imaging. 2013;**4**:199. DOI: 10.1007/s13244-012-0217-5

[46] Rosenblatt GS, Conlin MJ. Clipless management of the renal vein during hand-assist laparoscopic donor nephrectomy. BMC Urology. 2006;**6**:23

[47] Friedman AL, Peters TG, Jones KW, Boulware LE, Ratner LE. Fatal and nonfatal hemorrhagic complications of living kidney donation. Annals of Surgery. 2006;**243**:126-130

[48] Ahearn AJ, Posselt AM, Kang SM, Roberts JP, Freise CE. Experience with laparoscopic donor nephrectomy among more than 1000 cases: Low complication rates, despite more challenging cases. Archives of Surgery. 2011;**146**:859-864. [PMID: 21768434]. DOI: 10.1001/archsurg.2011.156

[49] Dekel Y, Mor E. Hem-o-lok clip dislodgment causing death of the donor after laparoscopic living donor nephrectomy. Transplantation. 2008;**86**:887

[50] U.S. Food & Drug Administration. Available from: https://www.fda.gov/ [Accessed: 27 July, 2018]

[51] Hsi RS, Ojogho ON, Baldwin DD. Analysis of techniques to secure the renal hilum during laparoscopic donor nephrectomy: Review of the FDA database. Urology. 2009;**74**:142-147

[52] Capocasale E, Iaria M, Vistoli F, et al. Incidence, diagnosis, and treatment of chylous leakage after laparoscopic live donor nephrectomy. Transplantation. 2012;**93**(1):82-86

[53] Box GN, Lee HJ, Abraham JB, et al. Comparative study of in vivo lymphatic sealing capability of the porcine thoracic duct using laparoscopic dissection devices. The Journal of Urology. 2009;**181**(1):387-391

[54] Kawamoto S, Fishman EK. MDCT angiography of living laparoscopic renal donors. Abdominal Imaging. 2006;**31**:361-373

[55] Sebastià C, Peri L, Salvador R, Buñesch L, Revuelta I, Alcaraz A, et al. Multi-detector CT of living renal donors: Lessons learned from surgeons. Radiographics. 2010;**30**:1875-1890

[56] Keller JE, Dolce CJ, Griffin D, Heniford BT, Kercher KW. Maximizing the donor pool: Use of right kidneys and kidneys with multiple arteries for live donor transplantation. Surgical Endoscopy. 2009;**23**:2327-2331. [PMID: 19263162]. DOI: 10.1007/s00464-009-0330-9

[57] Breda A, Bui MH, Liao JC, Schulam PG. Association of bowel rest and ketorolac analgesia with short hospital stay after laparoscopic donor nephrectomy. Urology. 2007;**69**(5):828-831. PMID: 17482915. DOI: 10.1016/j.urology.2007.01.083

[58] Wang J, Ma H, et al. Comparison of postoperative morphine requirements in renal donors and patients with renal carcinoma undergoing laparoscopic nephrectomy. Transplantation Proceedings. 2016;**48**(1):31-34

[59] Rege A, Leraas H, et al. Could the use of an enhanced recovery protocol in laparoscopic donor nephrectomy be an incentive for live kidney donation? Cureus. 2016;**8**(11). DOI: 10.7759/cureus.889

[60] Chin EH, Hazzan D, Herron DM, et al. Laparoscopic donor nephrectomy: Intraoperative safety, immediate morbidity, and delayed complications with 500 cases. Surgical Endoscopy. 2007;**21**:521-526

[61] Harper JD, Breda A, Leppert JT, Veale JL, Gritsch HA, Schulam PG. Experience with 750 consecutive laparoscopic donor nephrectomies—Is it time to use a standardized classification of complications? The Journal of Urology. 2010;**183**:1941-1946

[62] Jacobs SC, Cho E, Foster C, Liao P, Bartlett ST. Laparoscopic donor nephrectomy: The University of

Maryland 6-year experience. The Journal of Urology. 2004;**171**:47-51

[63] Mjoen G, Oyen O, Holdaas H, Midtvedt K, Line PD. Morbidity and mortality in 1022 consecutive living donor nephrectomies: Benefits of a living donor registry. Transplantation. 2009;**88**:1273-1279

[64] Boghossian T, Henri M, Dube S, Bendavid Y, Morin M. Laparoscopic nephrectomy donor death due to cerebral gas embolism in a specialized transplant center: Risk zero does not exist. Transplantation. 2005;**79**:258-259

[65] Jalali M, Rahmani S, Joyce AD, Cartledge JJ, Lewis MH, Ahmad N. Laparoscopic donor nephrectomy: An increasingly common cause for testicular pain and swelling. Annals of the Royal College of Surgeons of England. 2012;**94**:407-410. DOI: 10.1308 /003588412X13171221592177

[66] Shafizadeh SF, Daily PP, Baliga P, et al. Chylous ascites secondary to laparoscopic donor nephrectomy. Urology. 2002;**60**(2):345

[67] Reese PP, Feldman HI, McBride MA, Anderson K, Asch DA, Bloom RD. Substantial variation in the acceptance of medically complex live kidney donors across US renal transplant centers. American Journal of Transplantation. 2008;**8**:2062-2070. [PMID: 18727695]. DOI: 10.1111/j.1600-6143.2008.02361

[68] Nogueira JM, Weir MR, Jacobs S, Breault D, Klassen D, Evans DA, et al. A study of renal outcomes in obese living kidney donors. Transplantation. 2010;**90**:993-999. [PMID: 20844468]. DOI: 10.1097/TP.0b013e3181f6a058

[69] Lipkin G, Fenton A, Montgomery E, Nightingale P, Peters M, Wroe C. Age and gender-specific normal range for GFR in over 2500 potential UK live kidney donors; implications for selection and outcomes of live kidney donors. https://bts.org.uk/wp-content/ uploads/2016/09/BTS_Abstract_ pdf_2016.pdf

[70] Mjoen G, Hallan S, Hartmann A, et al. Long-term risks for kidney donors. Kidney International. 2014;**86**:162-167

[71] Muzaale AD, Massie AB, Wang MC, et al. Risk of end-stage renal disease following live kidney donation. Journal of the American Medical Association. 2014;**311**:579-586

[72] Ibrahim HN et al. Long-term consequences of kidney donation. The New England Journal of Medicine. 2009;**360**(5):459-469

[73] Boudville N, Prasad GV, Knoll G, Donor Nephrectomy Outcomes Research (DONOR) Network, et al. Meta-analysis: Risk for hypertension in living kidney donors. Annals of Internal Medicine. 2006;**145**:185-196

[74] Garg AX, Prasad GV, Thiessen-Philbrook HR, et al. Cardiovascular disease and hypertension risk in living kidney donors: An analysis of health administrative data in Ontario, Canada. Transplantation. 2008;**86**:399-406

[75] Textor SC, Taler SJ, Driscoll N, et al. Blood pressure and renal function after kidney donation from hypertensive living kidney donors. Transplantation. 2004;**78**:276-282

[76] Sofue T, Unui M, Hara T, et al. Short-term prognosis of living-donor kidney transplantation from hypertensive donors with high-normal albuminuria. Transplantation. 2015;**97**:104-110

[77] Fehrman-Ekholm I, Norden G, Lennerling A, et al. Incidence of end stage renal disease among live kidney donors. Transplantation. 2006;**82**:1646-1648

Chapter 4

Preoperative Assessment of Functioning Benign Adrenocortical Tumors: A Clinical Surgical Approach

Bruno Costa do Prado, Alana Rocha Puppim,
Jose Tadeu Carvalho Martins, Fabiana Lima Marques,
Robson Dettman Jarske
and Octavio Meneghelli Galvão Gonçalves

Abstract

In assisting a patient with adrenocortical tumors, the main concern is to establish whether the lesion consists of a malignant neoplasm and if there is any hormonal functioning, which are two instances that generally demand surgery. In distinguishing benign from malignant lesions, two aspects are particularly important: the size of the lesion and the image findings. In order to establish whether a lesion is hormonally functioning, it is necessary to carry out thorough clinical and endocrine assessments. The extension of such assessments is still controversial. This present chapter revises fundamental aspects of the propaedeutic of such tumors. Most guidelines agree that lesions smaller than 1 cm need not be investigated. The diagnostic and therapeutic approach of adrenocortical tumors imposes a difficult and challenging dilemma in terms of its approach, as it may be a benign finding or it may imply a high level of morbidity and mortality due to its hormonal activity or a possible malignant histology.

Keywords: adrenocortical tumors, adenoma, adrenal, Cushing's syndrome, aldosteronoma

1. Introduction

Adrenal gland tumors are common entities in clinical practice. They are divided as functioning (which produces hormones) and the nonfunctioning ones (also known as silent). In terms of their biological behavior, they may be divided in benign or malignant tumors. The term "incidentaloma" refers to adrenal masses that are found in image exams aiming at investigating disturbances unrelated to the adrenal glands [1–3].

Most adrenocortical tumors are benign, unilateral, nonfunctioning adenomas with less than 4 cm in diameter that are found during abdominal image studies [3]. The functioning adrenal tumors are generally the benign adenoma type, which cause, for instance, the Cushing's syndrome, primary aldosteronism, or, not so commonly, virilization [1, 2].

This present chapter discusses the preoperative assessment of patients suffering from this condition. It mainly focuses on:

1. Whether there is hormonal production by the tumor and the controlling techniques

2. The malignancy risk and the staging for propaedeutic planning purposes

2. Epidemiology

The frequency of adrenocortical tumor diagnosis has increased nowadays due to larger availability of image examination techniques, which makes it a relatively common clinical problem currently. Some studies claim a detection rate of 4% in all abdominal computer tomography [4]. Studies in series of autopsies identified that adrenal masses count less than 1% in individuals younger than 30 years of age and that the rate increases to 7% in those who were 70 or older [1, 2].

Adrenocortical tumors are more common in white, obese, diabetic, and hypertensive individuals. These data might be biased, as elderly, white individuals constitute the groups that most frequently undergo image examinations. It is known that such tumors are rather uncommon in individuals under 50 years of age and are especially uncommon in children [2]. They are more common on the right side [2, 3].

In terms of hormonal production, even though most tumors are nonfunctioning, in up to 15% of cases, there might be a slightly increased production of certain hormones, being cortisol the most common one, which may cause Cushing's syndrome [1].

Around 10–15% of all tumors found are bilateral [2]. Bilateral functioning adrenocortical masses may be congenital adrenal hyperplasia due to a 21-hydroxylase deficiency, adrenal macronodular hyperplasia, or primary hyperaldosteronism [2].

The most common causes of bilateral nonfunctioning adrenal masses are metastases, infections (mycosis, tuberculosis), lymphomas, bleedings, amyloidosis, and, rather rarely, carcinoma and myelolipomas [1].

In a decreasing order of occurrence, the adrenocortical tumor categories are:

1. Nonfunctioning adenomas (43–75%)

2. Cortisol-producing adenomas (including subclinical Cushing's syndrome) (10–15%)

3. Myelolipomas (6–8%)

4. Adrenal carcinomas (4–11%)

5. Metastatic lesions (3–10%)

6. Aldosteronomas (2–6%)

7. Cyst (5%)

8. Tuberculosis and lymphomas (3–8%)

3. Natural history

Natural history of adrenocortical tumors is still not completely known [1]. Some studies suggest that most incidentalomas remain within stable size for many years [2]. Long-term follow-up studies suggest that from 5 to 20% of cases involving tumors larger than 1 cm, there is an increase in adrenal mass after an average period of 4 years, regardless of the state of adrenal hormonal production [1]. The typical increase rate of an adrenocortical carcinoma exceeds 2 cm per year, with a survival expectation lower than 50% within 5 years [1, 2].

Occasionally, tumor reduction might be observed (3–4% of cases). Appearance of mass at the contralateral gland might also be noticed. Nonetheless, the risk of malignancy development is low (<1/1000) [1].

There is a risk that a nonfunctioning adenoma starts to produce some hormone during follow-up, especially if the mass is larger than 3 cm and mainly in the case of cortisol production. Prospective studies show a 0.3% risk of a subclinical Cushing's syndrome development and a 0.2% chance of it turning into a pheochromocytoma. After a 3- to 4-year follow-up, such risk reaches a plateau that is to say the possibility that it would turn into a functioning one is low. Therefore, repetition of screening for functioning is only prescribed during the first 5 years of follow-up [2].

For the reasons explained here, rather small nodules (smaller than 1 cm) with a benign tomographic aspect need not be further investigated by image, as the benignity chance is high, whereas the risk of growth is low [2].

4. Pathological findings

Adrenal adenomas are generally encapsulated, have variable volume and weight, and in most cases have a diameter of 2–4 cm. In nonfunctioning tumors, clear cells of the fasciculate zone, filled with lipids (cholesterol), predominate microscopically, which gives the yellowish coloration. Functioning tumors are usually of varied colors, reddish-brown, with yellowish areas or striae, showing in microscopy the predominance of compact cells, associated with clear cell nests (**Figure 1**). Cortisol-producing adenomas are accompanied by hypotrophy of the adrenal cortex of the affected gland and the contralateral adrenal gland due to adrenocorticotropic hormone (ACTH) (suppression in contrast to aldosterone-producing adenomas in which this aspect is not observed) [3].

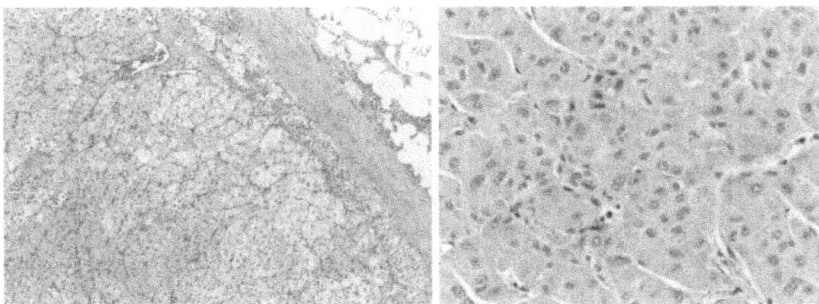

Figure 1.
Microscopy of an adrenal cortex adenoma showing one or more cell types (A) separated from each other by fibrous septa containing blood vessels (H&E 100×). High increase showing cells in the zona glomerulosa, fasciculate zone, and reticular zone forming nests and strands (H&E 400×).

Adrenal carcinomas are usually larger than 4 cm and occasionally weigh more than 1 kg. Microscopically, the picture is varied: in some cases, the tumor is very similar to the adenoma, but in some cases, the tumor appears anaplastically, being composed of cells with large pleomorphism, bizarre nuclei, and atypical mitoses. Vascular or capsular invasion is a predictive sign of malignant behavior, being a sign of local extension [3, 4].

Differentiation with adenomas can be difficult and is based on macroscopic (tumor weight, hemorrhage, and capsule integrity) and microscopic aspects using the modified Weiss scoring system. The five criteria used in the updated Weiss system include >6 mitoses/50 high potency fields, ≤25% clear tumor cells in the cytoplasm, abnormal mitoses, necrosis, and capsular invasion. Each criterion is scored 0 when absent or 2 for the first two criteria and 1 for the last three when present. The adrenal carcinoma can be diagnosed by the presence of a total score ≥ 3 [5].

Tumors are functioning in approximately 60% of all cases, but the presence of symptoms of hormonal hypersecretion is present in only 40%, possibly by the secretion of large quantities of biologically inactive hormones [5, 6].

In general, adrenal carcinomas rarely produce and secrete a single steroid hormone and are usually associated with overproduction and hypersecretion of multiple hormones and precursors. Most cases produce different types of steroid hormones [7–9]. Thus, hypersecretion of a single adrenocortical steroid usually indicates the benign nature of adrenocortical neoplasia. The most frequently seen combination is hypersecretion of cortisol and androgens [10].

5. Hormone assessment

There are basically three types of production by adrenocortical tumors:

1. Cortisol (corresponding to between 5 and 20% of cases)

2. Aldosterone (corresponding to 1% of cases)

3. Androgen (extremely rare)

5.1 Cortisol-producing tumors

Such tumors generally produce minute quantities of cortisol, which, most of times, do not suffice to increase the excretion of free cortisol in urine. They are, nonetheless, able to cause suppression of the hypothalamic-pituitary axis. Ordinarily, there are no Cushing-related manifestations in those patients. For that reason, this condition has been known as subclinical Cushing's syndrome or subclinical hypercortisolism [11]. There might be the classic Cushing's syndrome in long-evolving cases.

A suppression test with 1 mg of dexamethasone should be carried out at night for tracking Cushing's syndrome. The patient orally takes 1 mg of dexamethasone at 11:00 pm the night prior to sample collection of plasmatic cortisol, which is to be carried out at 8:00 am the following morning. Values that determine abnormal response of cortisol in this test varied in several studies from 1.8 to 5.0 mcg/dL, yet most guidelines lead to the following interpretation:

Levels of plasmatic cortisol <1.8 mcg/dL virtually exclude autonomous production of cortisol, with sensitivity >95% and specificity from 70 to 80%.

Cortisol levels between 1.8 and 5 mcg/dL have been considered to be undetermined.

Values >5 mcg/dL would indicate a highly probable diagnosis of Cushing's syndrome (specificity > 95%) [1].

An abnormal suppression of 1 mg of dexamethasone during the night is consistent with a positive tracking, and it should be confirmed by a 24-hour free urinary cortisol, which should then be followed by an investigation of the serum dosage of cortisol after a high dose (8 mg) of dexamethasone during the night and the serum dosage ACTH [3, 4]. This latter investigation aims at determining the origin of the Cushing's syndrome, as to refute a hypopituitary cause. This condition is typically presented with unsuppressed levels (ACTH dependent). For diagnosis of subclinical Cushing's syndrome, many experts propose confirmation under the following criteria:

Values > 5 mcg/dL in plasmatic cortisol at the 1 mg dexamethasone test without any other stigma

OR

At least two from the following results:

Levels of plasmatic ACTH < 10 pg/ml with an increased 24-hour free urinary cortisol and values > 3 mcg/dL of plasmatic cortisol at the 1 mg dexamethasone test [1]. **Figure 2** shows an algorithm of investigation of Cushing's syndrome.

Dehydroepiandrosterone sulfate is an adrenal androgen that is produced under stimulus of ACTH. Thus, an undetectable concentration of dehydroepiandrosterone sulfate in serum suggests a chronical suppression of ACTH levels [12].

Percentage of patients suffering from subclinical Cushing's syndrome that would evolve to the classic Cushing's syndrome is uncertain. It is estimated to be <1%, though [1].

Even though patients suffering from subclinical Cushing's syndrome do not present the classic stigmata related to hypercortisolism, they present, as suggested in some studies, in comparison with the population in general, higher occurrences of:

- Hypertension (40–90%)

- Type 2 diabetes mellitus or glucose intolerance (20–75%)

- Osteopenia/osteoporosis (40–50%)

- Hyperlipidemia (50%)

- Obesity (35–50%)

An increase in the carotid intima-media thickness has been recently reported, as well as alteration of coagulation parameters, decrease in the quality of life, and occurrences of mortality due to cardiovascular disease [1].

For those reasons, there is still no consensus about the approach to subclinical Cushing's syndrome. It may be treated clinically or through surgery [2].

Generally, in cases with many occurrences of comorbidity that might be attributed to hypercortisolism, such as systemic arterial hypertension, diabetes mellitus, dyslipidemia, osteoporosis, and central obesity, especially the ones that are difficult to control, a ponderation of the risk/benefit of surgical treatment by adrenalectomy of the affected adrenal should be carried out, as proposed for the treatment of classic Cushing's syndrome [2].

It is important to mention that up to 75% of patients might develop acute adrenal insufficiency (sometimes deadly) at the post-surgery phase of adrenalectomy in case they are not treated with glucocorticoid due to atrophy of the contralateral gland. This should be an additional functional endocrine characterization for the propaedeutic planning [1]. In case the adrenalectomy is carried out, there should be

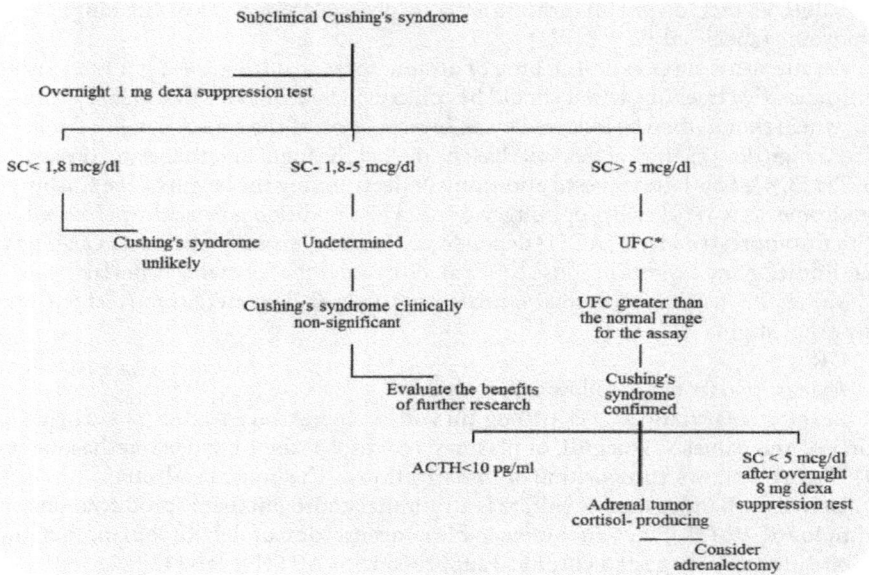

Figure 2.
*An algorithm for investigation of Cushing's syndrome in adrenal incidentalomas. Dexa, dexamethasone; SC, serum cortisol; UFC, urine-free cortisol; ACTH, adrenocorticotropic hormone. *At least two measurements.*

a perioperative coverage of glucocorticoid due to the risk of adrenal insufficiency, hemodynamic crisis, and death [12].

Weight loss, improvement of hypertension, glycemic control, and normalization of bone renewal markers are frequently found in the post unilateral adrenalectomy scenario of patients with subclinical or classic Cushing's syndrome [12].

5.2 Aldosterone-producing tumors

Also known as aldosteronomas, they are rare (less than 1% of cases), and their characteristic manifestation is systemic arterial hypertension associated with hypokalemia. Yet primary normocalcemic hyperaldosteronism is common (20–50% of cases) [1, 12]. For that reason, as most patients suffering from primary aldosteronism do not suffer from hypocalcemia, all patients suffering from hypertension and adrenal incidentaloma should be assessed through measurements of their aldosterone plasmatic concentration and plasma renin activity [12].

Initial endocrine investigation in such cases consists of dosing the levels of plasma aldosterone and plasma renin activity. In case the ratio between them is <27, the existence of hyperaldosteronism is virtually excluded. Other authors use further landmarks (between 20 and 30) to establish diagnosis as abnormal. Values >40–50 are almost hyperaldosteronism pathognomonic [1].

It is important to mention that if the laboratory can only assess the renin direct dosage (other than the plasma renin activity), the renin value must be divided by 12, so that the actual value of plasma renin activity is established, which will eventually be the one used for the ratio calculation. If the ratio is lower than 20, it can refute diagnosis. In case it is between 20 and 30, it indicates a likely diagnosis. Then, if it exceeds 30, with aldosterone dosage higher than 15 ng/dl, positive tracing should be considered and investigation should continue through tests for confirmation [2]. In patients with spontaneous hypokalemia, plasma renin below detection levels plus plasma aldosterone >20 ng/dL, it is suggested that there is no need for further confirmatory testing (**Figure 3**) [4].

The aldosterone and plasma renin activity relationship should never be used for patients under spironolactone, and in case doubtful results appear, other medications (a beta blocker, central alpha-adrenergic agonist, anti-inflammatory) that might cause a false increase of that relationship should ideally be suspended, as well as those drugs that cause a false reduction of the inhibitors of angiotensin-converting enzyme, aldosterone receptor blocker, thiazide, and dihydropyridine inhibitors of the calcium channel [2].

Patients older than 40 years of age suffering from confirmed hyperaldosteronism, even with evidence of adrenal images compactible with such diagnosis, should be submitted to adrenal catheterization for assessment of whether that increased aldosterone production is really due to incidentaloma or to adrenal hyperplasia, whereas the occurrence of nonfunctioning incidentalomas in the population older than 40 is no longer negligible (around 4%).

In such cases, adrenalectomy would not solve hormonal hyperproduction, which should be kept under control with the use of medication, aldosterone antagonists, such as spironolactone [2].

5.3 Androgen- and estrogen-producing tumors

In cases of congenital adrenal hyperplasia due to a 21-hydroxylase deficiency, it is rather common to find adrenal masses, either uni- or bilateral ones, presumably due to excessive chronic stimulation of adrenals by ACTH [1].

Sex-hormone-producing adrenal adenomas are very rare. Androgen-producing carcinomas are also uncommon. Nevertheless, patients generally manifest some virilization, which makes it unlikely for such tumors to be related to adrenal incidentalomas. Thus, the routine testosterone and estradiol dosage are not recommended for patients with adrenocortical incidentalomas who present trace of

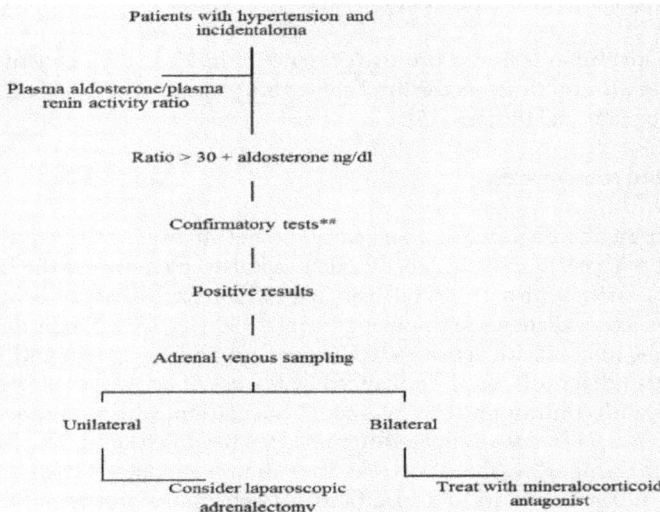

Figure 3.
*Algorithm for investigation of hyperaldosteronism in adrenal incidentalomas. *Most commonly used confirmatory tests: oral sodium loading test and intravenous saline infusion test. *In patients with spontaneous hypokalemia, plasma renin below detection levels plus plasma aldosterone > 20 ng/dl, it is suggested that there is no need for further confirmatory testing.*

virilization [1]. For individuals that present such virilization or high concentrations of androgens, adrenalectomy may be indicated for controlling of hormones.

Estrogen-producing tumors are rare and they are generally malignant. In men, it may manifest through feminization with gynecomastia, decrease in libido, atrophy of testicles, whereas in women, it could manifest through breast sensitivity and bleedings [12]. In such cases, adrenalectomy may also be indicated.

6. Adrenal image

As previously mentioned, most adrenocortical tumors are benign, nonfunctioning adenomas that were incidentally found in abdominal image examinations such as computed tomography and abdomen magnetic resonance imaging.

Adrenal incidentalomas rarely have a malign cause in patients with no known record of cancer. It is estimated that only 2–5% of incidentalomas are formed by adrenal adenocarcinomas, and around 0.7–2.5% of cases are caused by metastasis from tumors elsewhere toward the adrenal [13, 14].

Size and some other radiology characteristics of the computed tomography and magnetic resonance imaging might help differentiating an adrenal benign lesion from a malign one, with consequent perioperative implications. Adrenal tumors with surgical indication are generally approached through laparoscopy. On the other hand, in cases when an adrenal adenocarcinoma is suspected, open surgery is preferable, especially for larger lesions (>10 cm), or for those that might expand to other organs [15].

There is a direct relationship between the size of the adrenal tumor and the potential for malignancy. Average size of an adrenal adenocarcinoma at diagnosis is 10–11 cm, whereas most benign adrenal tumors present a diameter smaller than 5 cm [16].

Besides their larger size, malign adrenal tumors, in most cases, show on image exams as heterogeneous lesions, with irregular margins, suggestive calcifications, and a peripheral enhancement by intravenous contrast due to the core of the necrosis. Expansion toward other organs and lymph node involvement confirm malignancy.

Adrenal adenomas feature a profuse presence of lipids in their constitution. It is, therefore, very useful to assess the lipid contents by means of density calculation for differentiating adrenal tumors [15].

6.1 Computed tomography

The computed tomography is a very important exam in assessing adrenal tumors. At the phase with no contrast, a density calculus is used by means of the Hounsfield units (UH). Lesions with a <10 UH density have a high probability of being benign, whereas most adrenal adenocarcinomas present a >30 UH, which indicates low lipid content. Thus, tumors with density >10 UH demand further assessment.

Precision of diagnosis may be enhanced by the use of late stages of computed tomography with contrast and the "washout" calculation, which represents the fraction of contrast that is eliminated 10 min after administration. The finding of an average absolute "washout" of 50% after 10 min of contrast used in studies evidenced a 100% sensitivity and specificity for detection of adenomas in relation to adenocarcinomas, pheochromocytoma, and extra-adrenal metastases [17, 18].

All patients likely to be suffering from an adrenal adenocarcinoma should undergo a computed tomography of the thorax prior to surgery as any findings related to metastasis may alter the approach of treatment.

6.2 Magnetic resonance imaging

Despite the fact that the computed tomography is the most important exam in assessing adrenal nodules, in some situations it is imperative to resort to a magnetic resonance imaging.

Analysis of conventional images weighted at T1 and T2 is the most frequently used technique. Adrenal adenocarcinomas present an isointense sign in relation to the T1 liver and enhanced intensity of sign at weighted sequences at T2 (**Figure 4**). Typically, they present as large lesions (>5.0 cm) at the moment of the diagnosis and may include necrosis, bleeding, and, frequently, calcification [19].

After administration of gadolinium, a slight increase of sign is noticed, as well as a swift washout of contrast, whereas malign lesions present a fast and striking increase of sign followed by a rather slow washout pattern [20].

Chemical shift imaging is a detection technique for the presence of lipids. Benign lesions show as relatively shiny at the in-phase images, and they present a dimmed sign at the out-of-phase ones. The majority of adenomas are slightly hypointense or isointense to the liver on T1-weighted images and slightly hyperintense or isointense on T2-weighted images. The utilization of chemical shift techniques (in-phase or out-of-phase GRE) allows the characterization of adenomas containing microscopic fat and water protons in a same voxel (**Figure 5**). On out-of-phase images, the protons signal is null and results in signal loss as compared with in-phase images [21–24].

A magnetic resonance imaging may be superior to a computed tomography in the assessment of the vascular invasion, especially in terms of the inferior vena cava [25, 26].

6.3 Other resources of diagnosis per image

In patients whose characterization of lesion malignancy could not be carried out by a tomography or resonance, additional information could be obtained through fluorine-18 fluorodeoxyglucose positron emission tomography. Malignant lesions present a high collection rate of the radiotracer.

Metomidate binds itself specifically to Cyp11b cortical adrenal enzymes. It is used as a radiotracer at C-MTO PET, as it is capable of differentiating lesions originated at the adrenal cortical from the metastatic ones toward the adrenal [27].

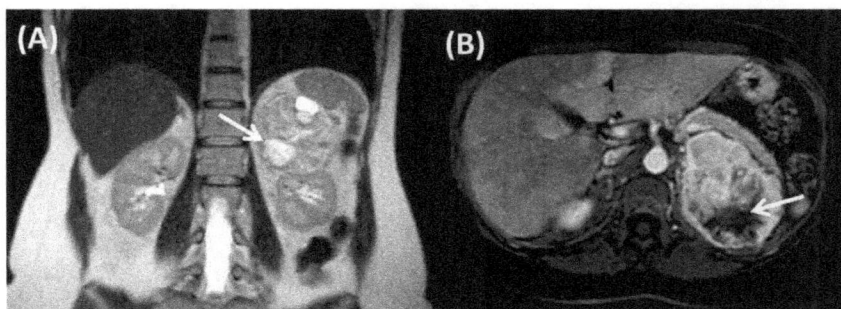

Figure 4.
Adrenal cortical carcinoma. Magnetic resonance imaging coronal T2-weighted FSE (A) and contrast-enhanced axial T1-weighted GRE (B) sequences demonstrate a large expansive lesion involving the right adrenal gland. The lesion shows heterogeneous pattern of impregnation by the contrast agent and areas of necrosis (hypersignal on T2-weighted sequences) (arrows).

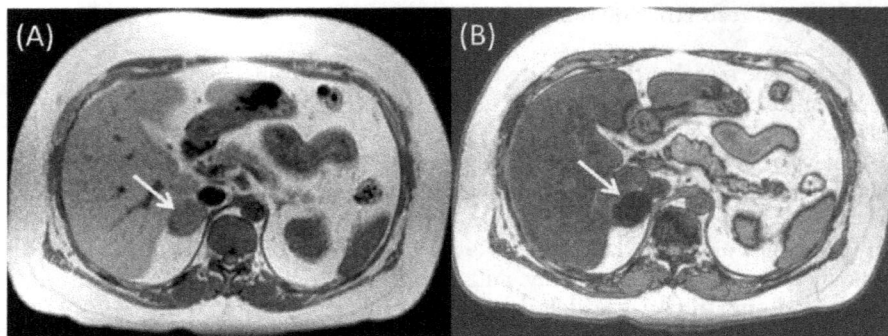

Figure 5.
Magnetic resonance imaging axial T1-weighted phase GRE (A) and axial out-of-phase sequences (B) demonstrate right adrenal lesions signal loss (arrows), allowing the diagnosis of microscopic lipid-rich adenoma.

7. Conclusion

Patients diagnosed with adrenal lesions should undergo a thorough assessment of functioning in light of the possibility of malignancy.

Functioning adrenal tumors or those likely to be malignant should lead to surgical treatment.

Special care should be taken in preparation prior to adrenalectomy of patients that might suffer from functioning tumors or pheochromocytoma.

Conflict of interest

None of the authors have any conflict of interest.

Abbreviations

ACTH	adrenocorticotropic hormone
UH	Hounsfield units
H&E	hematoxylin and eosin
SC	serum cortisol
UFC	urine-free cortisol
FSE	fast spin echo
GRE	gradient echo

Author details

Bruno Costa do Prado[1*], Alana Rocha Puppim[2], Jose Tadeu Carvalho Martins[2],
Fabiana Lima Marques[2], Robson Dettman Jarske[1]
and Octavio Meneghelli Galvão Gonçalves[3]

1 Department of Urology, Universidade Federal do Espírito Santo [Espírito Santo
Federal University], Vitória (ES), Brazil

2 Department of Clinical Medicine, Universidade de Vila Velha [Vila Velha
University], Vila Velha (ES), Brazil

3 Department of Radiology, Universidade Federal do Espírito Santo [Espírito Santo
Federal University], Vitória (ES), Brazil

*Address all correspondence to: brunocostadoprado@gmail.com

IntechOpen

References

[1] Vilar L. Manuseio dos Incidentalomas Adrenais. In: Vilar L, editor. Endocrinologia Clínica. 6th ed. Rio de Janeiro: Guanabara Koogan; 2016. pp. 621-649

[2] Sales P, Santomauro A, Cunha Silva M, Pires P, Alvarenga T, Pereira Marcon L. Incidentaloma Adrenal. In: Sales P, Halpern A, Cercato C, ed. by. O essencial em Endocrinologia. 1st ed. Rio de Janeiro: Roca; 2016. p. 121 - 135

[3] Pittella JEH, Coutinho LMB, Hilbig A. Sistema endócrino. In: Brasileiro Filho G, editor. Bogliolo patologia. 8th ed. Rio de Janeiro: Grupo Gen - Guanabara Koogan; 2011. p. 1149

[4] Carroll TB, Aron DC, Findling JW, Tyrrell B. Glucocorticoids and adrenal androgens. In: Gardner DG, Shoback D, editors. Greenspan's Basic and Clinical Endocrinology. 10th ed. New York: McGraw-Hill; 2018. p. 328

[5] Aubert S, Wacrenier A, Leroy X, Devos P, Carnaille B, Proye C, et al. Weiss system revisited: A clinicopathologic and immunohistochemical study of 49 adrenocortical tumors. American Journal of Surgical Pathology. 2002;26(12):1612-1619

[6] Hough AJ, Hollifield JW, Page DL, Hartmann WH. Prognostic factors in adrenal cortical tumors. A mathematical analysis of clinical and morphologic data. American Journal of Clinical Pathology. 1979;72(3):390-399

[7] Ng L, Libertino JM. Adrenocortical carcinoma: Diagnosis, evaluation and treatment. Journal of Urology. 2003;169(1):5-11

[8] Wooten MD, King DK. Adrenal cortical carcinoma. Epidemiology and treatment with mitotane and a review of the literature. Cancer. 1993;72(11):3145-3155

[9] Icard P, Chapuis Y, Andreassian B, Bernard A, Proye C. Adrenocortical carcinoma in surgically treated patients: A retrospective study on 156 cases by the French Association of Endocrine Surgery. Surgery. 1992;112(6):972-979 discussion 9-80

[10] Nakamura Y, Yamazaki Y, Felizola SJ, Ise K, Morimoto R, Satoh F, et al. Adrenocortical carcinoma: Review of the pathologic features, production of adrenal steroids, and molecular pathogenesis. Endocrinology and Metabolism Clinics of North America. 2015;44(2):399-410

[11] Carroll TB, Aron DC, Findiling JW. Massa suprarrenal incidental. In: Gardner DG, Shoback D, editors. Endocrinologia Básica e Clínica de Greenspan. 10th ed. San Francisco: McGraw-Hill Education; 2017. pp. 324-325

[12] Stewart PM, Newell-Price JDC. The adrenal cortex. In: Melmed S, Polonsky KS, Reed Larsen P, Kronenberg HM, editors. Williams Textbook of Endocrinology. 13th ed. Philadelphia: Elsevier; 2016. pp. 490-555

[13] Young WF Jr. Clinical practice. The incidentally discovered adrenal mass. New England Journal of Medicine. 2007;356:601

[14] Terzolo M, Stigliano A, Chiodini I, et al. AME position statement on adrenal incidentaloma. European Journal of Endocrinology. 2011;164:851

[15] Zini L et al. Contemporary management of adrenocortical carcinoma. European Urology;60(5):1055-1065

[16] Grumbach MM, Biller BM, Braunstein GD, et al. Management of the clinically in apparent adrenal mass ("incidentaloma"). Annals of Internal Medicine. 2003;138:424-429

[17] Szolar DH, Korobkin M, Reittner P, et al. Adrenocortical carcinomas and adrenal pheochromocytomas: Mass and enhancement loss evaluation at delayed contrast-enhanced CT. Radiology. 2005;**234**:479

[18] Peña CS, Boland GW, Hahn PF, et al. Characterization of indeterminate (lipid-poor) adrenal masses: Use of washout characteristics at contrast-enhanced CT. Radiology. 2000;**217**:798

[19] Fishman EK, Deutch BM, Hartman DS, et al. Primary adrenocortical carcinoma: CT evaluation with clinical correlation. American Journal of Roentgenology. 1987;**148**:531-535

[20] Allolio B, Fassnacht M. Clinical review: Adrenocortical carcinoma— Clinical update. Journal of Clinical Endocrinology and Metabolism. 2006;**91**:2027-2037

[21] Israel GM, Krinsky GA. MR imaging of the kidneys and adrenal glands. Radiologic Clinics of North America. 2003;**41**:145-159

[22] Mitchell DG, Crovello M, Matteucci T, et al. Benign adrenocortical masses: Diagnosis with chemical shift MR imaging. Radiology. 1992;**185**:345-351

[23] Krestin GP. Genitourinary MR: Kidneys and adrenal glands. European Radiology. 1999;**9**:1705-1714

[24] Namimoto T, Yamashita Y, Mitsuzaki K, et al. Adrenal masses: Quantification of fat content with double-echo chemical shift in-phase and opposed-phase FLASH MR images for differentiation of adrenal adenomas. Radiology. 2001;**218**:642-646

[25] Hricak H, Amparo E, Fisher MR, Crooks L, Higgins CB. Abdominal venous system: Assessment using MR. Radiology. 1985;**156**:415-422

[26] Soler R, Rodríguez E, López MF, Marini M. MR imaging in inferior vena cava thrombosis. European Journal of Radiology. 1995;**19**:101-107

[27] Hennings J, Hellman P, Ahlström H, Sundin A. Computed tomography, magnetic resonance imaging and ^{11}C-metomidate positron emission tomography for evaluation of adrenal incidentalomas. European Journal of Radiology. 2009;**69**:314

Chapter 5

Prenatal Diagnosis and Management of Sacrococcygeal Teratomas

Anca Budusan, Horatiu Gocan and Roxana Popa-Stanila

Abstract

Sacrococcygeal teratomas (SCT) represents a group tumors deriving from the primordial germ cells. It is the most common tumor affecting neonates, with a female to male ratio of almost 4:1.78. SCT are either benign (mature) or malignant (immature) with different outcome. With advancements in ultrasonography, more SCT are diagnosed prenatally. magnetic resonance imaging (MRI) is more accurate in describing the intrapelvic and abdominal extent of the tumor. Most fetal teratomas could be managed by planned delivery and postnatal surgery. The earlier the diagnosis and surgical intervention, the better the prognosis. A complete surgical excision of the tumor is necessary, including coccygectomy, to prevent recurrence. At the time of birth, most lesions are benign and surgical resection can be accomplished with relatively low morbidity and mortality. Recurrence is reported as 2–35% in patients with immature teratomas, tumor spillage, incomplete resection or failure to remove the coccyx. A long-term follow-up is required for any urinary or bowel dysfunction.

Keywords: sacrococcygeal, teratomas, surgery, children, tumor

1. Introduction

Sacrococcygeal teratoma is the most common congenital neoplasm. The word "teratoma" is derived from the Greek word "teratos" meaning monster. The first reported case was described on a cuneiform tablet dated approximately 2000 BC. Advances in antenatal imaging have let to prenatal detection of most SCTs and may avoid early mortality. Delayed presentation and presence of malignant elements continue to be poor prognostic factors, while surgical goal remains complete resection.

2. Background

Although rare, SCT is the most common tumor of the fetus and the newborn, with a reported prevalence of 0.25–0.28:10,000 live births. With more advancements in US (ultrasonography), more SCT are diagnosed prenatally.

2.1 Etiology

SCT arises from pluripotent cells of Hense's node that is present/located anterior to coccyx, a remnant of the primitive streak in the coccygeal region. The primitive streak is a longitudinal ridge of ectodermal cells at the caudal end of the bilaminar embryonic disc. It consists of totipotent cells, which are able to transform into any type of cells. This structure determines the future craniocaudally axis of the embryo and demarcates the embryo into left and right halves. If totipotent cells of the primitive streak remain after the fourth week, these cells give rise to a SCT [1].

SCT is a relatively uncommon tumor affecting neonates, infants and children.

SCT represents a group of benign and malignant tumors deriving from the primordial germ cells. Pediatric germ cell tumors (GCTs) are neoplasms derived from primordial germ cells and may occur both inside the gonads and extragonadal organs. The five main histologic categories of GCTs are: dysgerminomas (in the ovary), seminomas (in the testes), teratomas, choriocarcinomas and endodermal sinus tumor (ESTS) or Yolk sac tumor. The most common site of extragonadal GCTs in the pediatric population is the sacrococcygeal region and the most common type are teratomas.

The sacrococcygeal region is the most frequent location for teratomas, but teratomas may occur in almost any organ, tending to develop more commonly in midline or paraxial location and can be observed from the brain (cephalad) to the coccyx (caudal). Less common sites are the mediastinum, testes, ovary, retroperitoneum, head [2, 3].

Females are affected more frequently with a female to male ratio of almost 4:1.78. SCT are either mature, immature or malignant, composed of embryonic elements. A mature SCT is a benign tumor containing only mature components, while immature SCT contains immature tissues. SCT that contains malignant elements are considered to be malignant tumors. Mature and immature teratomas are considered as benign tumors and may undergo malignant transformation. At birth, the great majority of SCTs are benign. They can manifest malignant transformation with advanced age.

They appear as cystic tumors or solid. The cystic may be filled with serous fluid, mucoid or sebaceous material, or even cerebrospinal fluid. Virtually any tissue can be present in a SCT. Neuroglial tissue, skin, respiratory and enteric epithelium cartilage, smooth muscle and striated muscle fibers are the most common elements found. Also bone, pancreatic tissue, choroid plexus and adrenal tissues are less commonly identified.

2.2 Classification

Size of a SCT (average 8 cm diameter, range 1–30 cm) does not predict its biological behavior. Altman et al. defined the size of SCT as follows:

Small: as 2–5 cm diameter

Moderate: 5–10 cm

Large: >10 cm.

Antenatal diagnosis is important to avoid complications during delivery. Fetal US and MRI are the mainstay of antenatal diagnosis of SCT. MRI is more accurate in describing the intrapelvic and abdominal extent of the tumor and provides more information on compression of adjacent organs. Prenatal assessment of the fetus is critical for counseling the parents and planning surgical options. Because of acoustic shadowing by the fetal pelvic bones, US cannot always define the extent of SCT. Fetal MRI has been successfully performed to evaluate anatomy, content and extent of the tumor, but just a few small cases series have been published yet.

SCT arise from the base of the coccyx and may continuously grow in the posterior direction forming an external protrusion, or in the anterior direction, dissecting and distorting surrounding structures such as the rectum, vagina and bladder, but without invading them. Based on this morphologic characteristic, Altman et al.

have been defined The American Academy of Pediatrics Surgical Section (APPSS) classification [3–5]:

Type I: predominantly external with minimal presacral component—45.8%

Type II: present externally, but with significant intrapelvic extension—34%

Type III: apparent externally but predominantly a pelvic mass extending into the abdomen—8.6%

Type IV: presacral mass with no external presentation—9.6%.

2.3 Histology

SCT are graded histologically as follows:

Grade 0—tumor contains only mature tissue

Grade 1—tumor contains rare foci of immature tissues

Grade 2—tumor contains moderate quantities of immature tissues

Grade 3—tumor contains large quantities of immature tissue with or without malignant yolk sac elements.

3. Diagnosis

3.1 Intrauterine diagnosis

The majority of SCT present between the 22nd and the 34th week of gestation. The diagnosis of SCT on routine US is associated with a greater than expected incidence of prenatal and perinatal complications. Close antenatal follow up is needed to optimize patient counselling and treatment in the presence of a completely solid tumor and the onset of polyhydramnios. A poor outcome is usually correlated with placentomegaly, cardiomegaly or non-immune hydrops fetalis.

3.2 Associated anomalies

Associated congenital malformations are observed in 12–15% of cases and occur more frequently with presacral tumors. The incidence of various congenital malformations associated with SCT ranges from 5 to 26%. Of these, anorectal and genital malformations are most commonly. A growing SCT during the first weeks of embryonic life will encroach between the layers of the cloacal membrane and prevent descent and fusion of the urorectal septum to the cloacal membrane, resulting in a high anorectal malformation with a rectourethral or rectovestibular fistula. The presence of SCT in the same period of time (47th weeks), when cloaca is subdivided by the urorectal septum to form the anorectal canal and the primitive urogenital sinus, could prevent fusion of the genital folds, resulting in a bifid scrotum or hypospadias. The most commonly observed anorectal defects are: imperforate anus, anorectal stenosis and common vertebral anomalies are: sacral hemivertebrae, absence of the sacrum and coccyx [6].

Other associated anomalies include spinal dysraphism, sacral agenesis, dislocation of the hips and meningocele. Rarely, gastrointestinal or cardiac defects are associated with SCT.

Currarino triad represents association of anorectal malformation, sacral dysplasia and presacral mass. Delay in diagnosis of the presacral lesion is common because a rectal examination may not be possible in many cases with anorectal stenosis. Presenting symptoms in some of these unusual cases include perirectal abscess or fistula in ano (**Figure 1**).

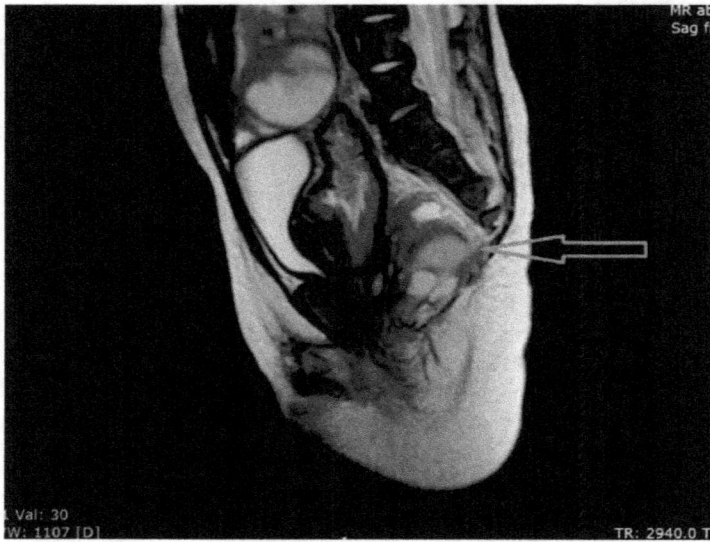

Figure 1.
Currarino triad in a female patient with SCT—MRI. Red arrow points the SCT. The girl presented with imperforate anus, recto-vestibular fistula and SCT was misdiagnosed until MRI.

3.3 Clinical presentation

Most external tumors are asymptomatic, with the exception of the presence of a visible exophytic large mass at the sacral region with occasional surface ulceration and hemorrhage and with anus displaced anteriorly (**Figure 2**). Sometimes, rupture of the tumor may occur as a result of a difficult delivery. Pelvic tumors or tumors that extend into the abdominal cavity may present with compression of the rectum or recto-sigmoid and urinary tract obstruction (constipation, frequent stools, obstruction of the bladder neck).

3.4 Diagnostic tools

Except for clinical examination, there are a variety of radiographic studies that can help. Plain X-Ray may show the presence of calcification within the tumor and anterior displacement of the rectum by the tumor. The sacrum may appear abnormal (such as hemivertebrae, agenesis).

Computer tomography (CT) or MRI of the pelvis with intravenous contrast material may reveal urinary tract displacement or obstruction and outlines the extent of the tumor more accurately. MRI is also a useful diagnosis of spinal cord extension of tumor (**Figure 3**).

A chest X-Ray or CT thoracic scan is obtaining to rule out the presence of pulmonary metastases.

Malignant SCT may have elevated tumor markers. The most commonly produced tumor marker is AFP (alpha-fetoprotein) because yolk sac components are the most common malignant elements. Other malignant elements may produce beta HCG (human chorionic gonadotropin). Serum AFP and beta HCG should be evaluated at the initial diagnostic work-up and assessed to monitor tumor relapse during the follow up period. The use of AFP as a tumor marker is well established and persistent, elevated level may indicate a residual tumor, recurrence or malignant degeneration. Because AFP is produced by fetal liver and fetal gastrointestinal tract,

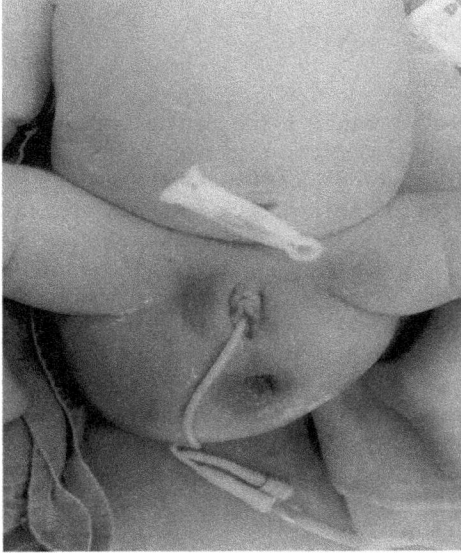

Figure 2.
SCT type II in a newborn girl. Large mass visible in sacral region, with displacement of anal orifice.

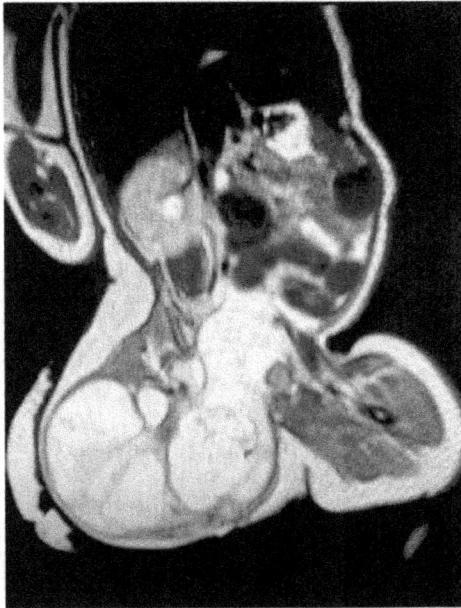

Figure 3.
Type II SCT with intrapelvic component—MRI.

its level is normally elevated in the first 8 months of life and after that age it rapidly falls to normal adult level (10 ng/ml). The mean time required for AFP to normalize after SCT resection is about 9 months [7, 8].

The differential diagnosis of SCT include rectal duplication, meningocele, lipoma, chordoma, epidermoid cyst, neuroblastoma.

4. Management

4.1 Prenatal management

Fetal MRI is a powerful addition to the prenatal evaluation of fetuses with SCT. Due to the fact that, in most cases, neonatal surgery is required soon after cesarean section, the anatomic details of tumor extent and involvement of adjacent structures may affect the surgical approach. Patients with significant intrapelvic extension of the tumor may need a combined abdominoperineal approach to control the blood supply and achieve complete resection. All these may contribute to avoid resection-related complications during surgery [9] (**Figure 4**).

Monitoring for fetal distress during pregnancy is very important. Some large tumors have a very high blood flow that causes a shift in blood flow away, producing fetal hydrops. Other possible complications are bleeding inside the tumor, polyhydramnios and preterm labor. A rare condition is called "mirror syndrome" where the mother mirrors the baby's sickness, leading to fluid retention, preeclampsia, high blood pressure, heart failure [10, 11].

4.2 Surgical management

Most fetal teratomas could be managed by planned delivery and postnatal surgery. The earlier the diagnosis and surgical intervention, the better the prognosis. A complete surgical excision of the tumor including coccygectomy is necessary, in order to avoid recurrence. A long term observation and follow-up is required for any urinary or bowel dysfunction.

Mature teratomas should not recur, if complete surgical excision and coccygectomy were achieved properly. Recurrence is reported in literature, as 2–35%, in patients with immature teratomas operated after the age of 5 months and is related to tumor spillage or incomplete excision.

At the time of birth, most lesions are benign and surgical resection can be accomplished with relatively low morbidity and mortality. The incidence of

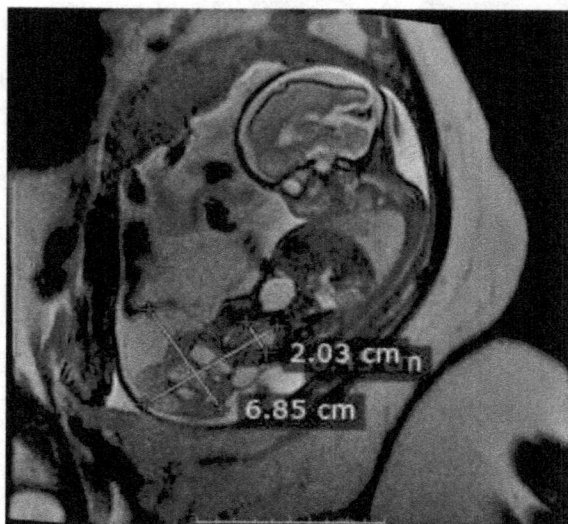

Figure 4.
Antenatal diagnosis of SCT using MRI and measurements.

malignancy in SCT is increasing with age. Failure to remove the coccyx results in 30–40% recurrence rate, with a higher probability of malignancy. Alpha fetoprotein may be used to detect early occurrence of malignancy.

Management of SCT depends on fetal lung maturation and presence of placental enlargement and/or fetal hydrops. When maturity of fetal lung without placental enlargement and/or hydrops fetalis, planned cesarean section is indicated. Some authors recommend preventive early delivery by cesarean section when the tumor exceeds the diameter of 5 cm, to avoid complications such as rupture and hemorrhage. The primary treatment of SCT is early surgical resection with complete excision of the coccyx. Early surgical intervention is associated with better prognosis. The surgical approach depends on the degree of pelvic extension. Posterior sacral approach is recommended in type I and II, and combined abdominal and posterior sacral approaches in type III and IV. The technique of wide resection of benign lesions with coccygectomy is helpful in preventing recurrence and has changed little over the last four decades.

The goals of surgical resection of an SCT are:

- Complete resection of the tumor

- Removal of the coccyx

- Reconstruction of the pelvic floor and ano-rectal sphincter

- Acceptable cosmetic appearance

After inserting a urinary catheter, the patient is placed in the prone jack-knife position. A V-shaped incision is made at the superior margin of the tumor. It is important to identify the course of the anus by placing a tube in the anal canal. After raising skin flaps, the muscles are dissected from the tumor which must be resected with the coccyx, after ligation of its main blood supply, which are middle sacral artery or branches from the hypogastric arteries [4, 7, 12].

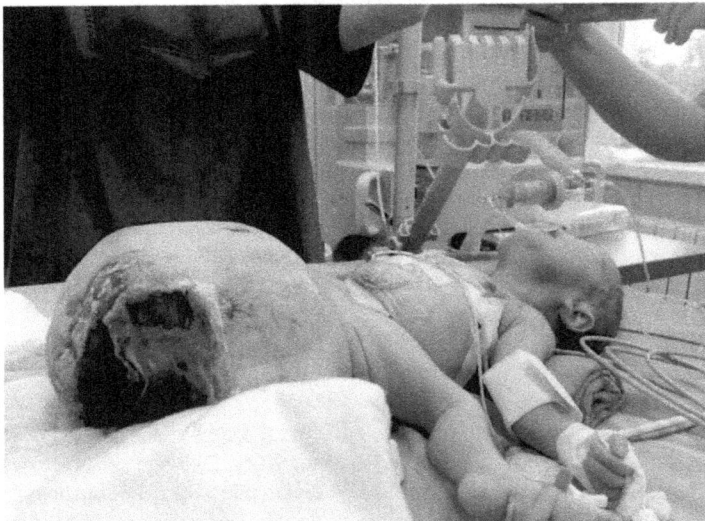

Figure 5.
Large SCT in a newborn—preoperative. SCT represents more than 50% of birthweight, with visible ulceration of the skin.

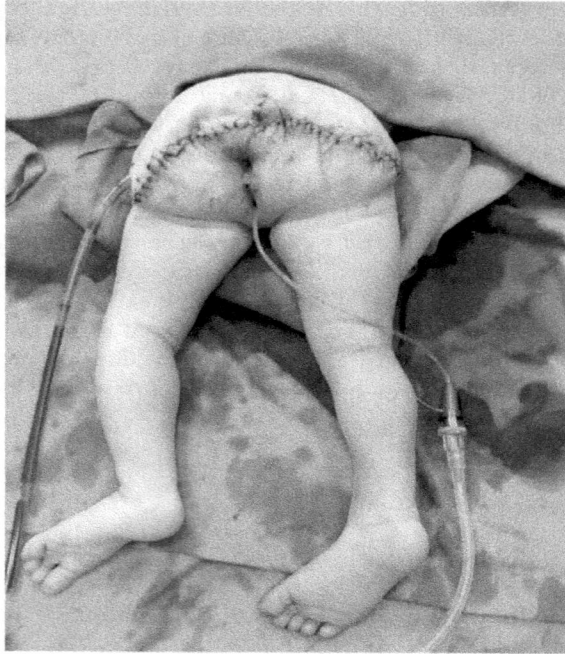

Figure 6.
Same newborn—postoperative view, after removal of SCT.

The multiorgan involvement makes the anesthetic management challenging. Prematurity and hypothermia are risk factors for coagulopathy and can lead to fatal consequences. Management of intraoperative bleeding and early extubation are good outcome predictors [5, 13, 14] (**Figure 5**).

Patients with malignant SCT are managed after surgery with irradiation if residual disease is present, and chemotherapy. Most tumors have a plane of dissection and can be removed easily. It is safer and recommended to catheterize the bladder to keep it away from the tumor and place a large rubber catheter in rectum for identification. Levator ani muscles are often stretched over tumor and should be reconstructed after tumor is excised. Drainage is necessary as there is a large raw area and collections should be avoided (**Figure 6**).

Preservation of the autonomous nerve supply to the bladder and rectum may be difficult. Therefore, postoperative complications (31%) that may be expected are bladder dysfunction, incontinence for feces and dysesthesia. The main postoperative early complication is wound infection because of the proximity to the anus and the skin flaps that may be needed.

5. Conclusions

SCT is a common neonatal neoplasm. Antenatal diagnosis is essential, for avoiding complications and high morbidity, mortality. Delivery in a tertiary center by cesarean section, when needed, should be emphasized. Early diagnosis and complete resection of the tumor with removal of the coccyx is associated with good prognosis.

Author details

Anca Budusan[1,2]*, Horatiu Gocan[1,2] and Roxana Popa-Stanila[1,2]

1 University of Medicine Cluj-Napoca, Romania

2 Emergency Children's Hospital Cluj, Romania

*Address all correspondence to: anca21b@yahoo.com

IntechOpen

References

[1] Bedabrata M, Chhanda D, Moumita S, Kumar SA, Madhumita M, Biswanath M. An epidemiological review of sacrococcygeal teratomas over five years in a tertiary care hospital. Indian Journal of Medical and Paediatric Oncology. 2018;**39**:4-7

[2] Szyllo K, Lesnik N. Sacrococcygeal teratomas—Case report and review of the literature. American Journal of Case Reports. 2013;**14**:1-5

[3] Niramis R, Anuntkosol M, Buranakitjaroen V, Tongsin A, Mahatharadol V, Poocharoen W, et al. Long-term outcomes of sacrococcygeal germ cell tumors in infancy and childhood. Surgery Research and Practice; 2015. Article ID 398549

[4] Hashish A, Fayad H, Ashraf El-attar A, Radwan M, Ismael K, Ashour M, et al. Sacrococcygeal teratoma: Management and outcomes. Annals of Pediatric Surgery. 2009;**5**(2):119-125

[5] Tuladhar R, Patole SK, Whitehall JS. Sacroccocygeal teratomas in the perinatal period. Postgraduate Medical Journal. 2000;**76**:754-759

[6] Alalfy M et al. Review article: Prenatal diagnosis and management of sacrococcygeal teratomas, a review of literature. Obstetrics & Gynecology International Journal. 2019;**10**(1):47-49

[7] Hussam S, Elbatarny A. Sacrcoccygeal teratoma: Management and outcomes. Annals of Pediatric Surgery. 2014;**10**:72-77

[8] Yoon HM, Byeon S, Hwang J, Kim JR, Jung A, Lee JS, et al. Sacrococcygeal teratomas in newborns: A comprehensive review for the radiologist. Acta Radiologica. 2018;**59**(2):236-246

[9] Danzer E, Hubbard A, Hedrick H, Johnson M, Wilson RD, Howell L, et al. Diagnosis and characterization of fetal SCT with prenatal MRI. American Journal of Roentgenology. 2006;**187**:W350-W356. DOI: 10.2214/ AJR.05.0152

[10] Girwalkar-Bagle A, Thatte WS, Gulia P. Sacrococcygeal teratomas: A case report and a review of literature. Anesthesiology, Pain Management, Intensive Care. 2014;**18**(4):449-451

[11] Calaminus G, Schneider DT, Bokkerink JP, Gadner H, Harms D, Willers R, et al. Prognostic value of tumor size, metastases, extension into bone, and increased tumor marker in children with malignant sacrococcygeal germ cell tumors: A prospective evaluation of 71 patients treated in the German cooperative protocols Maligne Keimelltumoren (MAKEI) 83/86 and MAKEI 89. Journal of Clinical Oncology. 2003;**21**:781-786

[12] Phi Phong N, Liem TT, DatHuy N. Sacrococcygeal teratoma in newborn: 4 cases had surgery at Danang Woman and Children Hospital. The Open Access Journal of Surgery. 2016;**1**:4-8. OAJS. MS.ID.555566

[13] Partridge EA, Canning D, Long C, Perenteau W, Hedrick H, Adzick NS, et al. Urologic and anorectal complications of sacrococcygeal teratomas: Prenatal and postnatal predictors. Journal of Pediatric Suregry. 2014;**49**:139-143

[14] Choudhury S, Kaur M, Pandey M, Jain A. Anaesthetic management of sacrococcygeal teratomas in infant. Indian Journal of Anaesthesia. 2016;**60**(5):374-375